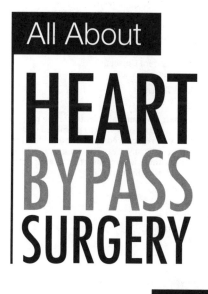

All About

HEART
BYPASS
SURGERY

Richard Trahair

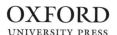

OXFORD
UNIVERSITY PRESS

OXFORD
UNIVERSITY PRESS

253 Normanby Road, South Melbourne, Victoria 3205, Australia

Oxford University Press is a department of the University of Oxford.
It furthers the University's objective of excellence in research, scholarship,
and education by publishing worldwide in

Oxford New York

Auckland Bangkok Buenos Aires Cape Town Chennai
Dar es Salaam Delhi Hong Kong Istanbul Karachi Kolkata
Kuala Lumpur Madrid Melbourne Mexico City Mumbai Nairobi
São Paulo Shanghai Singapore Taipei Tokyo Toronto

with an associated company in Berlin

OXFORD is a trade mark of Oxford University Press
in the UK and in certain other countries

National Library of Australia
Cataloguing-in-Publication data:

Trahair, Richard C. S.

All about heart bypass surgery.

Bibliography
Includes index.
ISBN 0 19 551305 3.

1. Coronary artery bypass—Popular works. I. Title.
617.412

Edited by Ruth Siems
Indexed by Richard Trahair
Text designed by Anitra Blackford
Cover designed by Racheal Stines
Typeset by Kerry Cooke
Printed through Bookpac Production Services, Singapore

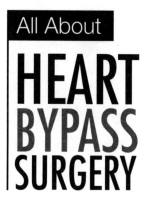

All About

HEART
BYPASS
SURGERY

Contents

	List of figures	vi
	Acknowledgments	vii
	Introduction	ix
1	Fourteen hearts	1
2	Why me?	14
3	'It's just *when* you have it done—there's no *if*'	27
4	In hospital before the operation	35
5	Having the operation	44
6	In Intensive Care	53
7	Complications after the operation	61
8	In the ward—later recovery	71
9	Rehabilitation	76
10	Life after a bypass	81
11	Challenges, recovery rate and advice	92
12	Later discomfort and problems	102
13	Conclusions and recommendations	110
	Glossary	115
	Selected reading	125
	Index	127

Figures

Figure 1   The heart and the circulation of the blood   15
Figure 2   The heart's arteries   17
Figure 3   What happens in a heart bypass   21

Acknowledgments

Many friends helped me find people who were willing to talk about their heart trouble and heart bypass operation. Also acquaintances in various branches of medicine helped me find a way to present technical matters on the heart so that it did not overwhelm the patients' stories and was sufficiently informative and relevant to the bypass operation and recovery in hospital.

Transcripts of interviews were typed by a medical secretary, Heather Eather, to whom I am most grateful for her patient and accurate work. I had great help from Geoff O'Callaghan and Ben Sandars in getting the project under way. Special thanks are due to the American Heart Association, Australian Cardiac Rehabilitation Association, Australian Institute of Health and Welfare, the Borchardt Library reference staff at La Trobe University, and the National Heart Foundation in Australia.

I am especially grateful to Peter Alsberg, Susan Berry, Ian Brett, Geoff Brown, Bess Carter, Cedar Court Cardiac Unit Staff, Carolyn De Silva, Carol Dobbin, Cathryn Game, Desmond and Kaye Gaunt, Heather Fawcett, David Harper, Richard Harper, Geoff Kinsey, Barbara McDonald, Bernard Newsome, Russ Newton, Anne O'Callaghan, David Petts, Michael Pontifex, Elizabeth Poynter, Richard Read, Peter Rose, Ruth Siems, Max Smith, Mitchell and Susan Smith, Les Tanner, Barlow and Sarah Telford, Ian Thorogood, Susan Trahair, Gill Tucker, and John and Sue Warburton.

I thank my fourteen informants, all of whom had at least one bypass operation. For each of them I chose a pseudonym as we agreed.

Introduction

This book is for people who are about to have heart bypass surgery, those who have just been through the ordeal, and those who are to care for a bypass patient. Based on the experience of fourteen informants, the book tells of life before the operation, the decision to have heart bypass surgery, preparation for hospital life, and recovery afterwards. It blends the patient's widely differing experiences with the surgeon's expectations, advice and technical demands, and the work of nurses, physiotherapists, occupational therapists, and other paramedical experts in the recovery from heart surgery.

Most people are shocked by the thought that they must have heart bypass surgery. While some feel resigned to their fate, others put on a heroic front; sadness engulfs a few, others are relieved to know what their ailment is, and some become angry. Most want to know why. As a rule, the cost of surgery and hospitalisation is not important to them. They want to know if they are going to survive. Patients who have private medical insurance find this operation costs them very little, and the conditions under which they recover in hospital are first class. In an emergency, few options are available to patients who need cardiac surgery; a surgeon will be chosen or recommended to you, and that surgeon will probably decide which hospital will be used. If you have no medical insurance, and your case is urgent, the operation will be done immediately, and usually the cost will be borne by the state. In the United Kingdom the cost is paid by the National Health Service or private insurance, although if you are not prepared to wait fourteen months, as reported recently, then the cost could be £10,000 for a quadruple bypass. In the United States costs vary depending on the insurance cover and the surgeon's fees. The total cost could be more than US$120,000, of which US$80,000 would go in hospital costs and the remainder to the surgeon and medical support.

Expect to be out of action for close to ten weeks. Most people spend a week in hospital and five to six weeks recovering at home and attending a rehabilitation centre. In some places you will not be permitted by law to drive a car for another two weeks. So allow two more weeks away from work, and be guided by your surgeon and cardiologist on what you can and should do.

Although there are signs and warnings of heart trouble, it seems that rarely do most people have much time to prepare for a heart bypass operation, and to make decisions about which surgeons and hospitals to employ. If you are not fully insured you will have your operation in a public hospital; if you have to wait for a bed, then your activities will be severely curtailed and closely supervised. If you are fully insured you will be operated on promptly and have some choice of surgeon, but probably the surgeon will decide which hospital you use.

The bypass operation itself is major surgery. It is such a shocking surgical procedure that as one of my younger informants said, 'You wouldn't want to know about it.' Under normal circumstances the operation takes about eight hours; you are well sedated before the operation, totally unconscious during the procedure, and afterwards spend about a day in an intensive care unit under close supervision. The physical shock to your body is enormous, but curiously enough the operation is not as frightening as you might think. Why? The decision to operate is swift, clear, and out of your hands; as one woman informant observed years later, 'Whatever goes on, it's better than the alternative!'

Because a full recovery can take many months, the recuperation is beset with frustrations. Notwithstanding, recovery is a joy to most sufferers of heart disease as the pain and discomfort ease, life with friends and relations becomes content, and happiness returns.

The recovery takes an unknown time, and its progress is often in your hands if no medical complications arise. There appears to be little you can do at first in preparing for the operation. If you are young and in good health recovery will be remarkably rapid and without strain. The natural fear and anxiety about the operation can be mastered easily by imagining the alternative.

But you can prepare for the recovery by anticipating and accepting that, for a surprisingly long time, you will not be the person you were before the operation; that you will feel a need to reschedule your life; that there are many new activities available and new skills to be acquired; and that professional help and personal care are readily available when you require them.

The book blends the experiences of patients with the expectations of medical experts. However, it is no substitute for medical advice. Pseudonyms are used to ensure confidentiality. All informants were uncertain about what to expect, shocked at finding they needed an operation, relatively ignorant of what they were in for, and highly dependent on the surgeon for a future. They included successful businessmen, mothers, an engineer, a hotelier, a surfer and fisherman, a lawyer, a travel consultant, a librarian, and a gardening and nursery manager, and they gave frank, articulate and careful thought to their stories of heart troubles, hospital life, rehabilitation, and recovery.

A glossary defines many of the medical terms in the text and selected readings tell readers what surgeons and paramedical staff do and expect from patients who have a heart bypass operation.

$$\textbf{1}$$

Fourteen hearts

The experience of heart trouble can be seen clearly in the following fourteen personal accounts leading to heart bypass surgery. The first group did not know their heart was diseased, and they were surprised to learn a bypass operation was needed.

These patients show signs of heart disease that are much like many everyday complaints, discomforts, and experiences, so it is tempting either to ignore them or to diagnose them to suit the needs of the moment. Sometimes it feels wrong to bother a doctor when the feelings are so trivial, and when it is so much trouble to seek medical information or advice.

Among the informants were some patients whose heart disease took a dramatic turn and brought great pain in different parts of the body, while others hardly felt anything that indicated to them that the heart was in trouble. Some informants recalled vividly and clearly the events that led up to their operation; others dismissed the serious symptoms, and considered them minor health matters that would not interest a doctor. Sometimes the signs appeared in the chest, sometimes in limbs and even down the throat. Among the informants were people who worried a lot about their health and felt often that their bodies were in trouble, while others hardly gave the signs a thought until serious symptoms appeared.

The conclusions are clear: for older people the signs of heart trouble are not always clearly evident until expert medical examinations have been done, and self-diagnosis is both inappropriate and life-threatening. Second, if you seek medical aid as soon as you can, then it is very likely that much distress associated with heart disease can be overcome.

'Would tomorrow suit you? We are doing a bypass'

David

David, in his early sixties, is a hotelier with many years of experience in related businesses. His father had his first heart attack in the late 1940s, and another in 1961. Each time he was told to lose weight and quit smoking. In 1964, feeling one hundred per cent, David's father resumed smoking, put on weight and, aged 56, died in 1970 of coronary occlusion. Knowing David's father well, David's father-in-law, a heart specialist, gave his son-in-law some advice.

> "He said, 'Don't smoke. Don't be overweight. Don't eat fatty foods.' And he said to stop smoking. 'You are going to die of a coronary occlusion like your father if you don't stop smoking, or if you put on any weight.' I said off-handedly, 'Yes, yes, yes.' I stopped smoking. And in 1984 I had my cholesterol tested and it was 7.2, and he said, 'You are still going to die of heart attack. Do something about it.' So he put me on Zocor tablets. I felt terrific. Nothing happened and nothing went wrong."

As a young man David played competition tennis and golf, travelled, and had climbed Uluru in Central Australia. But when he reached his early fifties, he would feel exhausted after a strenuous game of tennis.

> "With hindsight, when climbing Ayers Rock that time, and playing strenuous tennis I remembered getting indigestion. Not that it was bad, but the thought of it would keep me awake for an hour. I felt I was getting old."

After his father-in-law died, David's wife took on her late father's role.

> "'You haven't been for the tests that Dad said,' she warned. I went to hospital and had the walking test on a treadmill. They said, 'There's a glitch, but

it's not a problem.' I went straight back to the cardiologist and asked, 'What else is there I can I do? I've got to live with my wife. She told me I had to have these tests.' We did an angiogram. Afterwards he came to my bedside with the results. He asked, 'Would tomorrow suit you? We are doing a bypass, and we'd like to do it tomorrow. Some of your arteries are 80% blocked, some are 90% blocked.' I said I had a really important business meeting tomorrow. He said, 'Make it the next day.' So I had a quadruple bypass."

Rick

Rick, a successful businessman, had been a notable footballer and football coach in his youth. Like David, he had no indication that he would need heart bypass surgery. In 1980, aged 44, he came home from entertaining business clients. Feeling unwell, he blamed the cigars and fine port. After struggling through a sleepless night, and feeling clammy and short of breath, he went to the bathroom, bent over the basin and was suddenly dizzy. He was driven to a city hospital. In the emergency ward the medical staff sedated him, and he woke later in an intensive care unit, very tired. At the end of his bed stood an elderly lady.

"She asked, 'Do you smoke?' 'Yes I do.' She said, 'You know, if you didn't smoke, you wouldn't be in here.' She was the cleaner, standing there just as I came out of the dream. Her image stayed with me. I can tell you I've never had a cigarette since!"

Many tests were done in 1980 and he was sent to hospital for angiograms; results showed blockages in the blood vessels around his heart. He was advised to get fit, lower his cholesterol level and reduce stress. For him and his family it was a long, fifteen-year haul.

"And no smoking! The only problem was reducing cholesterol. We went on extremely strict diets under the watchful eye of this absolutely super cardiologist, got all the books, followed a low fat diet, and after nine months there was very little lowering of the cholesterol. Unfortunately I had one of those bodies that made a lot of cholesterol. So I had to go onto medication, Lipex, and I'm still on that today. That had a remarkable effect on the cholesterol. Now it hovers around 4.5 to 5, fairly satisfactory. We went for a long time, 1980 to 1996. In March 1996 I ended up having to have the zipper done."

Chris

Chris, who is retired, was amazed in his mid-fifties by indigestion and a chest pain that spread through his back. Unable to lie down, he would get out of bed, walk around the house, wave his arms, hitch his shoulders, and drink lemonade. The fizzy effect of lemonade staunched the pain. It was a minor discomfort. He did not want to know any more about it.

"These pains had happened about 1994 or 1995, and years later I even forgot to tell it to the cardiologist! It must be part of a defence mechanism to put aside things one doesn't want to record. Later I felt fine, quite normal, and all I wanted to do was work on the boat."

Two years later he was feeling off-colour and went for a medical check-up.

"Had the usual blood tests, listened to my heart, tapped my chest, did all the usual things for a general overhaul, and the doctor said, 'I can't find anything.' Perfect blood pressure. Maybe a bit high on the cholesterol level. Nothing to be concerned about."

Chris was varnishing his yacht one morning in October 1997. Holding onto the shroud with one hand, he leaned over the side of the boat to work on the nameplate.

"I got this amazing stabbing under my left ribs, like a stiletto driven into my back. If I hadn't been holding onto the shroud I would have fallen off the deck. Stood there for some minutes, got back to the cockpit, and breathed deeply to get rid of the huge indigestion pain. I didn't say anything to my wife. Thought it must have been some weird muscle spasm because I had twisted something."

Later he felt much better and decided to finish varnishing the boat.

"I said, 'I am going to finish this varnishing if it's the last thing I do.' Famous last words! It hit me again. Couldn't lift anything. But in two hours the pain had gone. Next morning I felt nothing was out of the ordinary. Then bang! I thought, 'I'm going to explode!' Lemonade! Staggered inside, rubbed my back on the interior walls, and brought relief with a few tiny burps from the lemonade. But as soon I stopped swigging the lemonade the pain came back."

He and his wife drove to the local doctor, who called an ambulance.

"Ambulance came in 10 minutes. Doctor had given me some tablets to dissolve under my tongue. In the ambulance paramedics gave me injections, saying, 'This will make you comfortable and stabilise you for the ten minute trip to hospital.' A woman doctor saw me in the emergency ward. Had an ECG, then a senior doctor said, 'If this had happened to you ten years ago, you'd be dead.'"

James

James is a university librarian and, like the others, had had no warning about the state of his heart, no indications that it might be diseased, and no discomfort other than a passing tiredness.

"A lot of people don't get *any* symptoms, they just have a heart attack and *that's it*. Ten years ago I just got tired walking to get to work, and I had to sit down when I got there. After a week my wife insisted I go to the doctor, who sent me to a specialist. He gave me an ECG and wasn't satisfied, and had me do a stress ECG on a treadmill in the afternoon at the hospital. He and the person operating the machine were very straight-faced. He asked me, 'How did you get here?' I said, 'Oh, I came by public transport'. Amazed, he turned to me. 'You're going straight into hospital this afternoon and I'll do an angioplasty. You've got private health insurance, haven't you?' I said, 'No.' He said, 'Well, you're very lucky because I'm the admitting officer of the hospital, I'll get you in tomorrow.' He did an angiogram and it showed two of my arteries were severely blocked and the third was going that way. He said, 'You know, there's a huge demand for bypass operations, and your case is not absolutely critical.' He gave me nitroglycerine tablets and I went home. Soon after I was hyperventilating, I was so anxious. Rushed to hospital, was in there for a few days and settled down. Because they still didn't have a vacancy I had the operation in a few weeks."

Peter

Peter had retired from business, became interested in hospital charities, and was helping his wife run her travel consultancy from their home in a seaside suburb. He had no warning of heart disease, and always thought health difficulties were of minor importance.

"Really had no problems. You could say that ten years ago occasionally I felt a bit tight round the throat. We were in the Pacific on Norfolk Island, climbing up a cliff near one of the two accessible beaches. I tend not to hang around, so I got to the top and I felt this pain at of the bottom of my throat. It was pretty uncomfortable, but only a bit of tightness. Not an awful lot."

Ethan

Ethan was one of a few soldiers who had survived a Japanese labour camp during World War II. On being repatriated he completed his law degree and practised in a large country town. There was nothing to indicate heart disease until, as he liked to tell, he was at golf, and was playing out of a bunker when he felt chest pain. He took little notice of it, until he felt its return when marching in the town parade later that year. His local doctor sent him to a specialist who gave him advice on what to do but Ethan did not follow the advice until, in 1989, chest pains returned.

His wife had a slightly different memory of the events.

"He was crossing the street one day in the town, and had a pain in his chest and down his arm. Immediately he went to the doctor. But knowing Ethan, the doctor, who was a friend, very cleverly sent him home straight away, and I put him to bed and he was not allowed to work for two months. That was well before he played that bunker shot."

Brad

Brad had established himself as a partner in a city law firm in the 1970s, and had been an active sportsman. Without any early experience of heart problems he had the first of *two* heart bypass operations.

"In 1980 I was walking to work in the city and I had a cold wind blow down my throat, no pain, no real discomfort. I saw a lung physician, who was astute enough to get me to see a cardiologist. Wasn't actually too worried because I didn't think that's what heart attacks were all about. I had a stress test at the hospital and that confirmed a heart problem. In 1981 I had bypass surgery. It was a week between seeing the cardiologist and then having the operation. Didn't work terribly well."

Hank

Hank is in his early forties, and lives outside a seaside township where he loves to surf, swim and fish. He had established a local business making surfing equipment, and invented equipment for surfers which became widely accepted in Asia and the United States. This had brought him business success. He married a nurse, and they had two daughters, now in their teens. In May 1996 his heart attack occurred without warning.

"After an argument with my daughter I had chest pains, pains I'd never had before, uncomfortable, so lay down, and they went away. Next day I was under a bit of stress at work, felt bad, and started getting pains after lunch. Effervescent sort of thing, that lasted only minutes, on and off, for an hour. The office girl insisted I went to the doctor. Drove to the next township, and I ended up having an ECG there. The doctor told me I was having an oesophageal reflux, a technical name for indigestion. I felt, 'Thank goodness. It's not the heart.' Went home, had a meal, another row with my daughter and got the same pain as the night before. Went and lay down again, thinking, 'It's not my heart. That's good.' The local doctor told me how to get rid of it with some stomach tablets. But it didn't go away. My wife looked at me, felt my pulse, and said, 'Hey, this is really bad.' She got the local doctor on the phone. The pain itself wasn't deep, it was debilitating, like there was someone holding me down on my back, and wringing me out like a dishcloth. I was sweaty and ended up taking all my clothes off, and just lying there, and feeling I wanted to go to the bathroom. The doctor came rushing up the stairs, started giving me some tablets, and I remember my wife saying, 'Just keep breathing.' I was thinking, 'If breathing is going to make this stop, I don't really care.' Later she said, 'That's the first sign of your body starting to shut down: when you begin to say to yourself, I don't care any more.'"

Hank learned that he had had a heart attack, was given more drugs and told that because he was so young and fit he would recover quickly. He had another heart attack, was classified 'unstable', and went to a city hospital where, after waiting two weeks before an angiogram was taken, he became most anxious to learn his fate.

"I was stressing out because no one could tell what was going on! Then I had an angiogram. I had 90 per cent blockages in two of my arteries. Two things they could do. Operate or wait."

Kim

Kim loved surfing, became a noted footballer and is an ebullient businessman. Following an interview for a management position with a large retail corporation, he had a few drinks with his friends, went home and felt ill.

> "Back in 1983 I had a pain in the left shoulder, it was stiff and I didn't feel that crash hot. My mother said, 'You've got to go to the doctor' and the doctor got me into hospital. I felt sick mentally. *I've* had a heart attack! I'm only *young*. I'm fit! I'm vibrant! I must be going to die! Dad died when he was young. I drove myself to hospital, walked in the door with a bag and said, 'Heart attack.' She said, 'Yes, where is he?' I said, 'I'm it.' She said, 'How did you get here?' I said, ' I drove here.' She got a chair and sat me down. In the cardiac ward they stuck tubes into me. Then I had another heart attack. It wasn't so much pain as a mental thing, right? People die with heart attacks, so automatically you lose confidence in your ability to recover. You get depressed, you say, 'I'm going to die. Right?'"

After four days in the intensive care unit, he began to feel better, was allowed to walk about the hospital ward, and was deemed fit enough to go home. Over the next fourteen years he took an aspirin daily, married twice, built two homes, refurbished others, raised six children, and never felt ill.

In 1997 he undertook the management of a large suburban market, and had just decided, amicably, with his wife, that within the next five months they would separate. Suddenly, he felt he was having a heart attack.

> "*Real* chest pain, not like the first attack, *real* pain. Woke up in the hospital casualty ward, they'd given me morphine, and I felt worse. Everything went peaceful, and I actually felt like I was lying on smooth stones under a babbling brook, looking up through the water, and could see the clouds going past, everything peaceful. And then I got zapped! I woke up with a man's thumb holding my mouth open, pushing in my top false teeth. And they're giving me a jump-start with electrodes! Bang! I was actually *dead*. My surgeon said, 'You know, you were actually gone.'"

The experience of dying led to Kim to offer the following advice to his friends. It summarises what can be learned from the experience of heart trouble.

> "I told all my friends, and I've got heaps of friends, if you get a pain in your chest or your shoulder that you don't understand, the first thing you do is you drive to a hospital and say, 'I think I may be having a heart attack.' It

costs you nothing, and I firmly believe if you're in a hospital they'll tell you whether you're having a heart attack, and you won't die."

Liam

Liam had retired as head of student counselling at his university. When young he had started a medical degree, and changed to psychology, married, joined the army, had children, and completed a postgraduate degree in clinical psychology before leaving the army. One night he was on his way home from the university when he felt something unfamiliar, and held a conversation with himself as he made his way home.

"Early in 1987 after work I was running late to catch a train. When I got to the top of the elevator I felt an iron band tightening around my chest. 'Oh, I can't do anything,' I said to myself, 'until I get to the bottom of this escalator. Started to ease off. Ah! now that's a good sign. Okay, this is not a clot, this is an angina attack. Just see if you can make it down to a train and get home, and proceed to seek medical help. Get to the platform, sit down. Rested, got my breath back.'"

After a comfortable night, next day he saw the university doctor who arranged a stress ECG, and prescribed Anginine tablets, to relax the blood vessels.

Later Liam had an angiogram. The specialist explained the results, and, concluding that a heart bypass was needed, explained the procedure in detail.

"For the angiogram they go into an artery in the thigh, put up this tube, none of which you feel, and you can actually watch the TV monitor and see the tube's movement. They warn you, saying, 'You'll feel a sensation of heat as we inject the dye now.' A sudden narrow band of heat moves across the chest, surges up and seems to bounce off the lower part of my jaw, and slowly dissipates. Not unpleasant, just unusual. On the TV monitor you can see the dye flow down the various coronary arteries. The doctor said there are three main arteries that provide nutrients to your heart, and the inner one on the right side is about 30 per cent blocked; that's quite acceptable at your age, but the main pumping artery that goes down the left ventricle, that's the one that keeps blood supplied to your brain, it's 90 per cent blocked. And the circumflex, which goes round to the back of the heart, is not so important, but nonetheless it gives a lot of nutrient to the heart, it's also 90 per cent blocked."

The specialist told Liam that for some patients whose blockage is limited, he could carry out an angioplasty, but in this case the narrowing went far down the blood vessel. That only left one option—bypass surgery.

"He explained all this in April 1987. Put me onto blood pressure lowering tablets, a tranquilliser, bed rest and I waited. If there were any dramatic symptoms, then I was to tell him straight away and it would be an emergency. My blood pressure lowered with tablets, I took life very quietly, doing nothing, watching TV, sleeping, didn't go to work at all and the operation was May 1987."

I knew the symptoms

The following informants had previous knowledge and experiences of heart disease, and were not surprised or shocked by the symptoms that indicated they would soon need the operation.

Lachlan

Lachlan is an academic in his late sixties. He studied philosophy and taught education, and recently retired after enduring the stress of administrative changes in university. In England during his late twenties he had learned about his diseased heart, but in hindsight, heart problems could have emerged earlier when, as a youth, he had applied without success to join the navy.

"I tried to join the navy as a cadet and was rejected on medical grounds. They kept on making me step up and down off a chair, and continuously listened with their stethoscopes. At the time they said nothing. I had an identifiable episode in England when I was 27. My wife thought it was a heart attack, and I was immediately rushed off to the doctor. Nothing wrong with me. I was a very good sportsman but I couldn't play squash. Absolutely exhausted after twenty minutes. So I already had incipient coronary artery trouble."

In 1985 his wife thought it would benefit him to mow the grass at home with a hand mower. The effort tired him. He believed that his weariness was due to smoking cigarettes. At the same time they were planning a trek through the Himalayas, and before going they had to have a medical check.

> "Our local doctor thought that we were healthy, and was very happy to sign the required medical document. He suggested that we go to our medical insurers, have a fitness check, and go on to a regimen of exercises so that we were *very* fit and would suffer less from altitude fever when we went up into the mountains. The medical insurers fixed us both up to a treadmill that made you walk very hard, and they had you wired up to a monitor. But they stopped my test and said that there was something wrong with me."

Signs of heart disease began to emerge rapidly. In June 1986 his medical report said that he was overweight, had high cholesterol levels and high blood pressure, and that, although his lungs functioned well, an ECG indicated blockages in his heart's arteries. Results of an angiogram showed Lachlan had only one half of one cardiac artery operating.

Catherine

In her fifties, Catherine had managed a plant nursery and florist business which often demanded long hours of work and placed sudden pressures on her. Family difficulties arose. She quit her business to care for her mother, who suffered with Alzheimer's disease. Suddenly her father died, and shortly afterwards her daughter's first baby died. Catherine's health was greatly affected at that time by congested heart failure related to a pulmonary embolism. After her heart failed she went into Intensive Care, and thereafter lived for twenty years with angina. It was controlled first with tablets and later more satisfactorily with a spray. Her health stabilised until early in 1999.

> "I had my grandson with me, put him to bed at about ten o'clock, and was watching TV when I had a little angina. I used my spray and half an hour later it came back. Next morning I phoned my daughter to say that I had problems and she should come over to pick up her son. I rang a friend and she took me to the doctor. I found out that I should've called an ambulance during the night. He put me straight into the ambulance and off to the local hospital for a few days. Then I was sent to a city hospital for angiograms and was operated on three days later."

Erik

Erik was born in Germany, and emigrated in the late 1930s. He became a metal worker, established a successful small business, and was noted for some valuable innovations and inventions. He is retired and lives by the sea, plays golf, and is a capable bridge player. In 1990 at a birthday party he became sick.

> "I felt indigestion. Before I went to the party I saw my doctor, who took an ECG and said, 'Maybe it's indigestion.' I couldn't eat a thing. Drank a brandy but I didn't feel any better so I drove home. At six in the morning I woke up and felt as though an elephant had put its foot on my chest. Couldn't breathe. I got to the phone, rang the emergency number. 'What's the problem?' I told them, 'I think I have a heart attack.' Within ten minutes two units came, they worked on me, took me to the local hospital and discovered I had a heart attack, an infarct. An artery had just crumbled."

Erik's heart was working well enough, and he was given drugs to strengthen the heart muscle. After twelve days he began a regimen of three-kilometre walks , a new diet, and Zocor to reduce cholesterol. He played golf regularly, and for five years had no health problems.

> "Then I noticed every time I start playing golf I get this funny feeling across the chest, as though my shirt was three times too small. It slowly wore off, but persisted at the beginning of every game for two or three holes. One day I got it even when I walked. And at night too while I'm playing a social game of bridge at home. No stress, no strain, no nothing. Also when I'm sitting down watching TV I get that pain again. I called the doctor and he said immediately to go to the hospital. In Intensive Care for a week, they stabilised me, and they tried to make me walk, but when I started I got that pain again. They sent me to the city hospital where they took an angiogram and discovered that I had three arteries blocked 80 per cent."

Barbara

Barbara is in her fifties, an occupational therapist, loves tennis, and has spent her married life raising a large family and supporting her husband in his duties as head of a boys' private school. Her children are grown up now. In 1988 she had angina, and a stress test showed minimal interference in the blood vessels. She felt well for two and

a half years, but at the back of her mind was the idea that she would
not live for long.

> "Running through my mind was an old phrase, 'I'm not going to make old
> bones'. We went abroad, and I was perfectly well. But I didn't want to walk
> up and down hills much. Lack of energy and enthusiasm. We were walking
> around the wall at Dbrovnik. I said to my husband, 'You go up. I'll just wait
> for you.' Feelings of not enough energy. No pain, nothing like that."

Early in 1991 after further bouts of angina, and feeling exhausted
on hot days, she found she did not even want to play tennis. When-
ever she moved she felt angina. Thinking that she was about to have
a heart attack, the school doctor sent her to the local hospital.

> "They wired me up, did blood tests, and said I hadn't had a heart attack. But
> in the middle of the night I had severe chest pain. They really worked on
> me, but it didn't pass, and they were obviously very anxious. Next morning
> the heart specialist came and said I was to go straight to a large city hos-
> pital. There they did an angiogram and said that the artery leading to the
> left side of my heart was all but blocked. They said if I walked out the
> hospital doors, they might not be able to get me back in time."

Why me?

Patients' experiences come in two groups: the first were unexpected emergencies, and a heart bypass operation had to be carried out as soon as possible; the second group had five or more years of heart trouble that eventually led to a bypass operation. Why did heart trouble come in different ways at different rates? If we look at what the heart is, what it does, and how it gets into trouble, the answers are clear.

The heart as a pump

The heart is a muscle with a right and left side that pumps blood around the body in a continuous flow; the right side pumps blood to the lungs, while the left side pumps it to the other parts of our body.

Each side has a pumping chamber (ventricle) and a priming chamber (atrium). The priming chamber fills the pumping chamber with blood, and thereby makes the heart pump work efficiently. This is done in three steps; blood flows into the atrium, the atrium fills the ventricle, and the ventricle forces the blood out of the heart around the body. So that the blood always flows in the same direction, there are four valves between the atriums and ventricles and between the main blood vessels to the heart and from the ventricles. The blood vessels are muscular tubes, quite elastic, known as arteries and veins. The arteries that take blood to the lungs are pulmonary arteries; the arteries that take blood to the rest of the body are

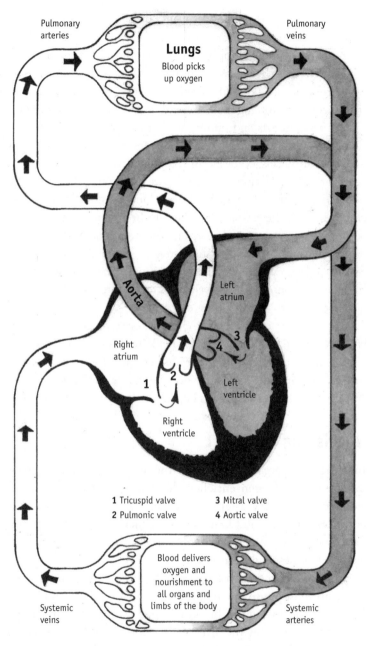

Note: Shaded areas indicate oxygenated (red) blood.

Figure 1: The heart and the circulation of blood

systemic arteries; the pulmonary veins take the blood from the lungs into the left side of the heart; the systemic veins take the blood from the limbs and organs of the body to the right side of the heart.

The heartbeat begins as an electrical discharge in clusters of cells in the right atrium (known collectively as the pacemaker). The right atrium contracts, forcing blood into the right ventricle. The right ventricle then contracts and pumps blood through the pulmonic valve along the pulmonary arteries into the lungs where the blood is filled with oxygen, necessary for life; the blood returns to the left side of the heart into the left atrium where it is pushed through the mitral valve into the left ventricle, which contracts and pushes the oxygenated blood through the aortic valve into all the systemic arteries of the body where it nourishes the organs and limbs. The blood leaves the organs and limbs by way of the systemic veins and enters the right atrium, and the cycle of blood flowing through the heart pump, arteries and veins continues. The cycle takes ten to fifteen seconds, and the heart beats ten to twenty times per cycle.

The heart is driven by an electrical system governed by the brain, which controls the heart rate. When the brain excites the heart—for example under stressful conditions—the heart rate surges, and when the stress abates the heart rate falls back to normal. As a rule the heart rate swings between 60 and 100 beats a minute.

Nourishing the heart

Like the other organs of the body, the heart also requires nourishment from the oxygen-enriched blood. Blood is taken to the heart along two coronary arteries—the right main and the left main coronary arteries—and branches from them. The left main coronary artery is short and has two branches, the circumflex, and the left anterior descending arteries.

All activities require a blood supply, some more than others, so the heart must pump much blood on some occasions, and little on others. As the amount of blood pumped through the arteries and veins varies, so does the size of the blood vessels. They enlarge when much blood is needed for vigorous activities, and contract when we are resting. The heart's coronary arteries need to be quite elastic to cope with great changes in our activities and to ensure that the muscle of the heart itself is well nourished.

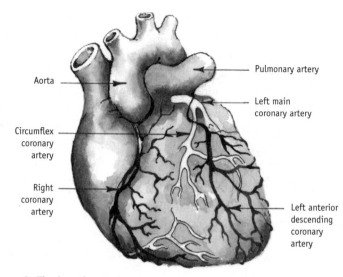

Figure 2: The heart's arteries

When heart trouble begins

The heart can become diseased in many ways, one of which involves the blocking of the coronary artery blood supply to the heart muscle. If the coronary arteries are narrowed and insufficient blood gets to the heart to meet the body's requirements, a heart attack can result.

In other forms of heart disease, the valves can fail or get so affected that the blood flow between the heart's chambers is impeded, or there can be a sudden change in the rate of pumping due to faulty electrical charges from the brain. However, it is heart disease resulting from problems with the coronary arteries that leads to a heart bypass.

A heart attack, or myocardial infarction, is caused primarily by atherosclerosis—the formation of fatty deposits in the arteries, often with associated hardening. The process of this 'hardening' of the coronary arteries is known as arteriosclerosis or coronary artery disease.

Fatty substances adhere to the walls of the coronary arteries, narrowing their diameter, and restricting the flow of nourishing blood to a stage where there is not enough blood available to keep that part of the heart alive. This can leave a dead spot in the heart muscle; but unlike our skin, the heart muscle cannot grow again. The death of that part of the muscle is a heart attack, and the pain of a heart attack is a result of the muscle spasm, as part of the heart dies. In some people, so much of the heart muscle is damaged during the convulsive shuddering that blood supply to vital organs, especially the brain, becomes inadequate, and they die.

The fatty substances begin building up when we are young, and when the rate of growth is maintained or spurts ahead rapidly our life is threatened, because it not only affects the heart muscle's blood supply, but also the blood supply to our intestines, kidneys, and brain.

Causes of heart disease

Advancing age, heredity, diabetes and gender are uncontrollable causes of heart trouble.

Usually we do not learn how clogged our arteries have become until late in life. This is why the longer one lives, the more likely it is that our arteries will clog with fatty deposits. So age is an important determinant of coronary heart disease. Heart disease also seems to run in families, so there is a heritable propensity for developing heart disease. Diabetes mellitus, an inherited disease, may in the long term contribute to arteriosclerosis of arteries.

More men than women have heart disease, although recent research shows the difference to be narrowing. Perhaps it is because more and more women are taking to cigarette smoking, which seriously threatens the heart's welfare. Perhaps taking replacement hormones after menopause limits women's chances of heart trouble because the therapy reduces blood cholesterol levels.

Controllable causes of heart disease are smoking, high blood fats, high blood pressure, overweight, lack of exercise, and stress.

Smoking not only damages the lining of the coronary arteries, but also limits the blood's capacity to take oxygen to the body's limbs and organs, and thereby helps considerably to promote heart trouble. High blood pressure, or hypertension, contributes to heart disease by wearing out the lining of the heart's arteries. Its cause is not securely known, but it is clear that when blood pressure is abnormally high, the heart must work excessively, and in doing so can damage the artery walls.

High levels of the wrong kind of blood fats or cholesterol in the blood make for an excess of fatty deposits on the artery walls. Also, if the body is not exercised regularly the number and size of collateral blood vessels may decline; then, if the heart's arteries are severely narrowed, there are too few reserve blood vessels to accept the work of supplying the heart with blood. Furthermore, regular exercise seems to help cut the build-up of fatty deposits on the artery wall by reducing the level of cholesterol in the bloodstream. It also seems that being 25 per cent overweight increases the risk of narrowing the coronary arteries.

Finally, leading a highly stressful life may add to the risk of heart disease. Some psychological research shows that among people who suffer from high stress there are more time-conscious people, who overwork compulsively (Type A)—than relaxed individuals, who work in an easygoing manner (Type B).

Given these observations, doctors tend to advise patients over 55 years—especially men—with a family history of heart disease, to quit smoking immediately, reduce cholesterol level with a change of diet, maintain the right weight, exercise regularly—walk or swim for 20–30 minutes three times a week—avoid stress, and have regular medical examinations for other controllable risks of heart trouble.

Warnings of heart disease

Warnings of heart disease require immediate medical attention. Heart trouble seems to follow an identifiable course in general, but is not easily predicted for any individual. So general warnings are based on family history and on daily habits that put our heart at risk. When the arteries narrow severely, then the oxygen supply to the heart muscle becomes inadequate and some people feel discomfort in their chest. Sometimes it is an unfamiliar crushing, squeezing feeling in the middle of the chest that often follows some exertion, and is relieved by rest. The feeling can spread from the centre of the chest, the breastbone, even to the neck or head, or towards the right or left arm, or down to the top part of the stomach. If you rest for fifteen minutes it might go away. This is the commonest indication of angina pectoris, and a sign there is a poor supply of blood to the heart muscle.

These indications require immediate medical attention, but they may not be due to what you suspect. They could indicate many disorders other than heart disease. If they do indicate angina, then it is not the end of life; your doctor will show you the appropriate treatment for a restricted flow of blood in a heart artery.

If the discomfort in the chest is anything from surprising to excruciating, and definitely moves to the left arm, or to the right in some cases, and you begin to perspire heavily, recognise indigestion that will not go away, feel sick, begin to vomit, go dizzy, feel faint or actually faint, and find rest no help, then get a doctor immediately. These symptoms point to a complete—not partial as with angina—blockage of an artery in the heart, and it may mean part of the heart muscle is going to die. Even if these symptoms appear mild, and you suspect—and do not want to think or imagine—that you are having a heart attack, then get emergency medical treatment. If treatment begins soon after the attack, then irreparable damage to the heart can be avoided.

Heart trouble as a process

So heart trouble in general is a gradual series of steps in ageing, a process that begins when we are young. Fatty deposits build up along the artery walls and limit the supply of nutritious, oxygen-rich blood to our heart muscle. At some time when we exert ourselves, because of the narrowing, or perhaps thrombosis (a blood clot), or a coronary artery spasm, insufficient blood flows through the restricted coronary artery, and, at worst, our heart muscle is permanently damaged. Immediate medical attention, and a period of professional treatment—or even heart surgery—can readily restore us to an acceptable life, not necessarily much different from life before the heart trouble.

For more than thirty years, coronary heart disease has been treated successfully with a coronary artery bypass graft operation. In this operation, an inessential vein and/or artery is sewn into the blocked blood vessel that nourishes the heart so that a detour is made around the obstructions. In some cases there can be two or three obstructions to be bypassed.

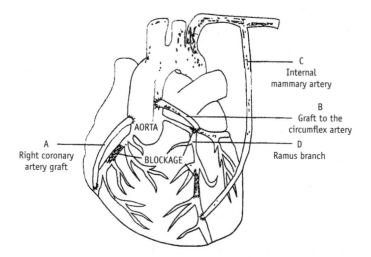

Figure 3: What happens in a heart bypass where 75 per cent or more of the blood flow is blocked. A and B are saphenous vein grafts from the leg; C comes from the mammary artery.

Why did I get heart disease?

Each informant had a different story to explain why heart trouble had happened to them. Barbara thought that being a chronic diabetic and eating fatty foods were the contributing factors to her heart trouble.

> "For thirty years I have been diabetic, but on insulin for only fifteen. That was contributing factor. Never smoked. Had a high-fat diet. I liked peanuts and they are 50 per cent fat. Used to eat cups of peanuts. That didn't help. My mother had cancer and died young, and her sister lived to 91. Her brother died of diabetes. It was diabetes and diet, although I was eating healthily."

Lachlan reconstructed the reasons for his need to have a bypass operation from what he had learned about his body, his history of apparent heart problems, the undeniable process of ageing, and giving up a poor health habit.

> "The capacity of my body to produce cholesterol is greater than normal. I have a hectic liver. Coronary heart disease is in my family: my mother had a heart attack when she was about 55. She didn't die until she was 91. If you've got it,

it will only get worse. I always had the belief that I was stronger than anything I might have. So I didn't worry about it. I went on vacation and immediately gave up smoking. That was an interesting experience. I'd given it up many times before with terrible side effects. On this final occasion absolutely none whatsoever. Didn't cough, didn't feel itchy, but I was not able to work."

He was at a newly established and poorly managed university college. His illness became the reason for giving up administrative duties, which he believed tended to 'damage to the people who are in it'.

Catherine's heavy smoking and a family history of heart disease, together with a high cholesterol level, promoted her heart trouble.

"I have always been slim and I've *tried* to put on weight. But that fattened up the arteries. My mother had high blood pressure and my father had his first heart attack at 50, but both lived until their eighties."

For twenty years she had heart trouble, and ate little except at celebrations. Shortly before her bypass operation early in 1999, Catherine had many stressful experiences. She had just divorced—the children were in their early to late twenties—and she was managing a florist and plant nursery that could easily become very heavy work. Suddenly everything bad happened at once.

"That was the year my parents died. My father was living in another state, and worried about my mother's Alzheimer's disease. I came down to care for her. I came on the Friday, she was admitted to hospital on Monday, and my father went to the hospital, rushed upstairs, got into Mother's ward, and he dropped dead. Tremendous shock. My mother died a lot later. On the day my father was buried my daughter lost her first baby. All contributed to the stress."

She was not angry or sad about the need for her bypass surgery. She understood the problem, and 'felt reassured, that I was facing major surgery, and it was for my benefit'.

Because his father had died from a cerebral haemorrhage at 72, Chris thought his own heart trouble was due to heredity. But he also felt he was certainly no candidate for heart disease if you looked at his everyday life.

"It's a hereditary thing. I'm not overweight, never smoked, not a diabetic, although my father had been one. I've drunk alcohol, of course. My last cholesterol reading was 5; my cardiologist wants me to get it down to 4. There's severe damage to my heart. It's working well, but I have to remember blood vessels leading into it are probably becoming progressively blocked with cholesterol and I could find myself back there on the surgeon's table."

Ethan's partner in their law firm died shortly after they had established the partnership, and Ethan carried the work load of two in a large, busy country town. Recognising the role of heredity in heart disease he recalled that his father had had angina and died at 72 in 1942. But Ethan also thought there were other reasons for his own heart disease.

"Smoking as much as anything. Being a prisoner of war under the Japanese could be a reason. But there was so little to eat most blood vessels would have had very little cholesterol in them. I smoked a pipe and was a medium cigarette smoker. Had no diabetes. Never been overweight. I am the same weight as I was when I was 20. I had diseases in the prisoner-of-war camp: paratyphoid, malaria, beriberi. The wet beriberi would have been the most likely to have affected my heart."

Rick had none of the feelings associated with heart trouble before he became ill in the mid–1980s. He was devoted to being fit, had recently finished coaching one of the nation's leading football teams, and had taken up the assistant coaching position at another. He felt as active as any of the young players. He had no thoughts at the time that the problem was one in the family. He believed that he became ill due to stress and to high cholesterol, after a heart attack at the age of 59, and well before he knew about the contribution of the history of family health to heart disease.

"There was discussion about stress. When I had the heart tests, my wife and I thought about stress. The question put to my wife was, 'When he's addressing the football players, coaching, do the veins on his neck stand out?' She said, 'It's more than the veins on his neck that stand out.' I had a high level of cholesterol. So positive action was taken. Lowering cholesterol with the right diet, giving up smoking. lowering stress, and we try to get supremely fit. No suggestion of diabetes. The major problem was high cholesterol. There was some degree of high blood pressure, but it never changed. It was the cholesterol. Strict diet. But it didn't work!"

David had had strong and persistent warnings from his father-in-law that he was a perfect candidate for heart trouble. So his major thoughts were not about the origins of his heart trouble, but the consequences of the treatment.

"Why me? I *knew* it was going to be me! But to counteract that—after you have a bypass you are whole! It's not as if you haven't got an arm, or you lose a leg. It was not really unexpected because of my family history, and because of my father-in-law saying that something was going to have to be done. He was right in everything medical."

In hospital, after the initial indicators showed he might have heart trouble, Hank was told the origins of heart disease. From the many causes, he preferred to emphasise a mixture of family history, smoking and cholesterol as the major contributors. Before the attack he had no clear knowledge of what the process had been, largely because he was young, and, like Rick, was remarkably fit, and had no thought of serious health problems.

"Why it happened was clear when they gave us all this diet information, and the reasons why people have heart attacks ... It was my family history, I was an ex-smoker, and I had very high cholesterol. I remember one of the old boys down at the local jetty, he'd had a bypass, saying how hard it is to recover if you are a smoker. I was never a heavy smoker, but I was an ex-smoker. And there was a bit of stress in it to. To educate us before going home they were saying, 'You can't continue to eat fatty food.' Dieticians gave talks. I was fully aware that I had high cholesterol *before* it happened. And I've been on a low fat diet for nine years."

Unlike Hank, Peter thought about his health. He believed he was very fit, but recalled that, two years before he discovered how serious his heart problem was, his elder brother had had an episode.

"After one of these marathon walks my brother ended up having a bypass. So I was made aware of the fact that I might be doing the same thing. I had it in my family. My father died of a stroke. I know when my mother died at 79 she had a slight heart problem."

Peter's doctor asked about smoking, noted that Peter enjoyed wine and spirits, and had him admit to eating an excess of cheese, and to exercising very little. Stress was the next issue.

"Our doctor had some idea of our lifestyle, and asked about stress. My first wife had died in 1983 of leukemia after a three-year illness. I remarried a year later. Our doctor was aware of stressful events round about that time. I was trying to establish a fishing business which failed unfortunately. That was very stressful for a couple of years. Doctor said to me, 'Look, it's 50 per cent you, and 50 per cent hereditary and there's not much you can do about it.'"

A senior cardiologist told Peter, who was planning a business trip to India with his wife, that he could have a heart problem due to high blood pressure.

"So I did a treadmill test, and it showed a bit of abnormality. I've always been really very fit. That didn't bother the cardiologist. He gave me pills and said that if I was in pain to take them. Freely admitting he didn't realise the extent of the problem he wanted to see me when I came back to have an angiogram. We went, came back, went to see him and he did the angiogram. You can see this little probe on a monitor wandering around over your heart. There's a blockage, and there's blockage, and there's another blockage. I didn't get terribly excited about all this. Then he made the comment that if he'd known how bad it was I wouldn't've gone to India."

Erik was not concerned about the need for his operation. He decided there was no family history of heart disease, and concluded that he simply did not know why he got heart disease.

"In my family, I know one grandfather died of thrombosis of the leg, which is a clot, and in those days that was a killer. My father died very young, but he died of leukaemia and my mother died of cancer. So it is not necessarily inherent. I just don't know."

Kim was well acquainted with the role of heredity in heart disease, and had learned that when signs of ill health appear you should get medical advice immediately. Also, he felt certain that in hospital he had actually died. However briefly, he had experienced the alternative to having a bypass operation. So he had gone well beyond asking the question 'Why me?' His father had died of a coronary occlusion, and in 1987 his brother had had a quadruple bypass.

"He's as fit as a young steer now. I didn't feel the anger of the question 'Why me?' What would I feel angry about? There was never anything happening. I'd never thought about having a heart attack. My dad died when I was young.

My brother had had a bypass, he laughed at my first heart attack. That's life. I could get hit by a truck crossing the road! Why me? You're dead!"

He recalled the sensation of his heart missing a beat like frequent breaks in an electrical circuit.

"I kept getting these sensations of ectopic heart beats, and electric charges were firing and they couldn't find why. The hospital registrar said, 'You've got the insides of an 18-year-old.' One day I had that sensation in hospital and I felt I was looking into a starry sky, and then I was all right again. A nurse came running in and she asked, 'Did you have the sensation a little while ago?' I said, 'Yes.' She said, 'You actually died. Your heart stopped beating for about seven seconds.' She was at the desk, and saw it happen on the monitor. Then they put a catheter into a blood vessel, and they go up into your heart—you're watching it on TV—and you have a local anaesthetic. They want to find where the circuits are breaking that make you get these irregular heart beats. They couldn't find it. I still get an irregular heart beat. When I really exert myself I can miss anywhere between the seventh and the thirteenth beat. 'That's just a short circuit,' I say, and I'm confident, and I feel good. Lot of people have it and they never know they have it. When I had the first heart attack I got pericarditis and I got a lot of scar tissue around my heart, and from then I've always had a higher heartbeat than normal. When I was young my heartbeat would be between 60 and 70. After the heart attack my heartbeat went up to 90 or 100. Now it's back to about 80 since I've had the bypass."

$$\textbf{3}$$

'It's just *when* you have it done— there's no *if'*

The decision to have bypass surgery is difficult because patients have so little time to prepare for the experience. After a close examination of blockages in cardiac arteries, the cardiologist, the surgeon and other doctors advise on a bypass operation. However, if you are asked to decide, on what grounds could you make the decision? Feelings about the need for the operation? The impression of the doctor who will perform the work? The hospital? These are non-medical grounds for a life-and-death decision. So how do patients get ready to make this decision?

From the patient's point of view, the surgeon is the leading adviser, and agreement to surgery is based on two factors: first, that there is no choice where imminent death is concerned; second, confidence in the surgeon and his colleagues.

Confidence in the surgeon is based on the surgeon's reputation among cardiologists, cardiac physicians and doctors to whom the surgeon is well known. Patient confidence also appears to be some-times based on a surgeon's personal appearance and manner, and on their interpersonal skills with the patient.

The skills that patients value centre on the clarity of the surgeon's explanation of the medical procedure, and the capacity to reply to questions that patients state vaguely and find emotionally difficult to frame. During the presentation of the technical procedure the patient is looking not only for an intelligible account of what will happen, but also for evidence that the surgeon can grasp and understand what dominates a patient's feelings, especially patient anxiety about life and death, and the pain after surgery. As he speaks with and listens to the patient, the surgeon is examined for the reliability of the medical procedure he will use and the trust that can be put into the empathy he has for the individual. Even if the surgeon is accepted on these three grounds, patients still hold a residue of distress. The surgeon is expected to show in some way that he can readily reduce tension with generally acceptable habits and styles of response such as wit, perhaps a little humour, even a little self-deprecation, softening the idealised image that the patient has been offered of him, and showing that he is, like the patient, at core a plain character of good will as well as one who is highly skilled at successful heart bypass operations.

Erik had confidence in his surgeon because of the man's reputation, informativeness, and appearance.

"I knew I would have the operation. I talked to the surgeon, asked him, 'Would you do it, please?' He now runs a major city hospital. He is young, very handsome ... I liked the way he made a graph of what we were going to do and showed me where it's blocked. And he wrote on the piece of paper: 98 per cent success, 2 per cent failure of such operations. No problems. I just felt confident."

David was told that the surgeon wanted to operate next day because two arteries were seriously blocked. This was a surprise because there was no indication of a heart problem from the test on the treadmill or the angiogram. David had no difficulty accepting the decision, because he might suddenly die as his father did. Also, he had the chance to think about the kind of person he was.

"I'm a fatalist, and when someone says, 'You've done this, and you've done well, and this is the end of the line,' well, nothing I can do about that. I don't worry about things I can't do anything about. If he had said to me, 'Look, you'll live for ten years if we don't do it. You might die if we don't do it,' then I'd have a problem. He just said, 'We've got to do it. Tomorrow would suit us.' When I think of my father, that decision was *fantastic*!"

David had previously joked with an old friend who was a surgeon, 'If I have a problem, you are going to have to look after me.' But this conversation went out of his mind during discussions with the cardiologist.

"When they told me I had to have the operation, the cardiologist asked, 'Do you know any surgeon to do the job?' I said that I didn't. The cardiologist said he would get somebody for me ... So when my old school friend came in, I put my hands over my eyes, and I said, 'You went completely out of my head!' He said, 'I'm happy ... You've got the best man for the job.'"

Hank thought for a while that he had a choice He wanted the least troublesome solution, but eventually found the decision taken from him, because, so he thought, of his age.

"They could give me an angioplasty or they could give me a bypass. It was a choice. I remember them asking me. With an angioplasty they are mucking around with your groin, and it's uncomfortable, and I can remember thinking, 'I would rather have a bypass because at least I wouldn't feel anything.' Finally *they* decided that I was going to have the bypass. My age did come into it. They said I was pretty young. I was worried, because if they sent me home I'm going to have a heart attack out at sea in the boat, and I'm going to die."

He was adequately informed about the operation itself, and the chances of success, and knew that since it was deemed an emergency, it would be done immediately in a public hospital.

"The cardiologist said that there is a risk that you can die. One per cent. 'You being as old as you are, halved that risk. Nothing to worry about.' The anaesthetist and the surgeon came, and someone else ... showed me the film, saying, 'You have to watch this film now. If you have any questions ask me about it.'"

Hank did have an important personal question. How competent was the surgeon chosen for him? Like most people, he knew no surgeons, and certainly had no technical knowledge to help make a choice. But he had to ask *someone*.

"The surgeon sat down ... and he asked, 'You got any questions?' And I said, 'Yes. You any good?' And he says, 'I'm *really* good. *The best.*' So I said, 'Take your time, and do a good job.' When I went to see him afterwards, he said, 'You weren't that guy who cracked that joke?' ... Turns out he *was* the top man!"

Brad's operation was no emergency. The decision was taken by Brad in conference with the cardiologist, who had recommended the surgeon. Brad was led to believe that the surgeon was well known, so the decision was based on reputation. The operation was done almost three months after the decision was taken.

"Discussions in January and February, and I was done in March 1981. He was *the man* at the time and he's still going twenty years after. I had to wait because it was done in a public hospital, why I don't know. Probably because the private hospitals in those days didn't have the facilities. My second heart operation was in 1990, for the same thing."

From an initial examination it was not clear that Ethan had heart trouble, so a specialist's opinion was sought. The local doctor had thought Ethan was suffering from indigestion. The heart specialist was in a small city nearby.

"He made me do a walking test on a treadmill and as a result he recommended I should have an operation."

Ethan's wife added important facts.

"He had a heart attack while on the treadmill, and was rushed by ambulance to the hospital for war veterans well north of the city, but unfortunately it was Easter and not much could be done. The specialist at the hospital said he should have an operation."

The local doctor recommended the surgeon, and Ethan did not get to know him at all.

"I had plenty of confidence in him. It was a decisive moment. 'Come along! Do this. See you at hospital on such and such a date.' And after the operation, 'You're all right. You can go home now.' He was not abrupt. He was decisive, businesslike. If I didn't do it I'd be in the grave, good and proper. No choice."

Chris had private health insurance and was no stranger to surgery. The local doctor asked what hospital he preferred, and assured him that the one he chose had an excellent cardiac unit. He had had a series of severe heart attacks, and the cardiologist wanted to stabilise him at the hospital, then send him home. She did not recommend surgery so soon after the heart attacks. Better for him to rest a week or more and then see if surgery were needed. He went home, and found he lacked the strength to do much.

"I walked as much as I could, and two days before the next appointment with the cardiologist when I was coming home from walking the dog, and I felt I was going to pass out, hung on to a telegraph pole for a couple of minutes, got home, told my wife."

His cardiologist said that he had to go back into the hospital immediately, otherwise he would die. It was grim advice, but came from a woman he had grown to admire.

"She is a marvellous person ... no pomposity, explains everything in every detail one wants, and explains it well. Immediately you feel, 'I'm safe.' She was *encouraging* in that either you have the operation or you die. She was also *encouraging* in her attitude, such a breezy character. Works the most amazing hours. Trust is very essential. If you don't trust the people involved your condition gets worse."

Peter was satisfied that his cardiologist had recommended the best available surgeon. Peter himself had no choice. He considered that was quite appropriate—after all, who was he to question a cardiologist's decision? Later Peter was mildly irritated to find that he had had three surgeons, not one.

"My cardiologist said, 'You're coming in after Christmas.' That was when the surgeon that he wanted me to use would be back from abroad. So I went into hospital January and had a quadruple bypass on the 4th. There the surgeon, one of the big boys, a professor, at the city hospital, popped in to say 'Good Day'. I saw him once, very briefly. My cardiologist chose him. I had no say in it. My cardiologist is a top cardiologist, one of the best, and if he says that surgeon is the best surgeon in the world, that will do. Who am I to query that? The other thing was there's actually three surgeons! You don't find that out till you come to pay."

Her doctor in the local hospital had told Barbara how ill she was. The monitoring of the heart attack she had in the early morning of the first night in hospital had shown there were serious problems, and she was taken immediately to a city hospital where her angiogram examination showed that the artery on the left side of her heart was all but blocked. Staff warned her that if she were to leave she would die. At the city hospital she was allocated to a physician and a surgeon, who told her she had to wait.

> "I got put on the operating list, and it was a week before I was operated on, 13 March 1991. I was in bed in the hospital, allowed to walk a little, but only on the heart surgery floor, carrying patches and a little hand-held machine."

Like Barbara and Peter, James had no choices at all. A medical friend helped him understand decision-making in hospitals and this was a comfort.

> "My cardiologist said there was absolutely no choice. It's just *when* you have it done. There's no *if*. My doctor referred me to the cardiologist, and then he referred me to his surgeon .... I felt very confident ... But if I didn't know it wouldn't have mattered because I had faith in the system. The city hospital is a huge public bureaucracy, and everything functions well. I felt happier with that, than going to a newly established little private hospital that's into making money. The public system has got the whole city's university facilities behind it, and an enormous reputation."

Lachlan's heart trouble had begun with angina in 1986. His blood pressure was stable, he monitored his diet, and thought exercise was not so important. But in May 1987 he discovered after a brief angina episode that he couldn't walk home easily, felt breathless, and had no energy. He had always been physically strong. The cardiologist planned the bypass operation.

> "The choice was made absolutely by him ... I had a good talk with the surgeon who operated on me ... All my doctors did a thorough job on my history and diagnoses."

Lachlan's experience led him to reflect on the politics of the relation between surgeons and cardiologists within the hospital system.

> "Cardiologists have a lot of power to organise within the hospital who does the operations and how they are to be done. I've discovered cardiologists have rights in some hospitals and not in others. My cardiologist had rights in a city private hospital where he did all his angiograms, and in a team of cardiologists at the city public hospital. He would've known that I was insured, so he could've sent me to the city private hospital, if he wanted to. The surgeon he chose for me was doing research on the operation. In 1987 it was a relatively new operation in *his* context. Now they've done so much research and have learned a lot about it. My surgeon's research in 1987 would've helped operating nowadays."

Lachlan had considerable respect for the competence of his medical advisers, and in the close relation between surgeon and patient. But at the same time he was to see himself a victim of the hospital's industrial relations.

"I think it makes a difference if you bond with your adviser. The adviser knows the circumstances, and that the operation has got to be done—now! Well, my operation wasn't done immediately, but within two weeks. They had a hospital strike! That meant no elective surgery. So my operation was delayed. My cardiologist told me to stop work, do a lot of walking, get as fit as I could before I had the procedure, and not worry. I liked that, *don't worry*!"

Liam, who was 59 at the time of his operation, had a good knowledge of heart trouble before he became a patient, and was impressed by the competence of his cardiac physician, who gave a detailed account of which blood vessels were blocked, and the various options relevant to his case.

"All that was left to me was to *be* at the operation! The surgeon and the cardiac physician came to the decision to operate in discussions with my general practitioner. The cardiac physician's told me which blood vessels were blocked and of the treatment options, and why an operation was needed."

Liam's cardiac physician recommended the surgeon at a suburban private hospital. The surgeon reviewed all his data, agreed to operate, and went through all the options that the clinical tests gave rise to.

"I had very great confidence in the investigation by the cardiac physician, also the surgeon, who was a cousin of my colleague at the university. A warm, empathic guy. He wasn't one of these cold know-alls who can anticipate most of the questions. He related very well person-to-person, and was very open to discuss everything. I felt considerable confidence, particularly as it was backed up by reports I later received from various people about him. One said, 'I'd trust him with my life and I'd certainly trust him with yours.'"

Liam then accessed an informal group of medical acquaintances who told more about the surgeon. Impressions of the surgeon were most important.

"In explaining the operation my surgeon said that naturally you're apprehensive, it's a major, lengthy operation, but the risks nowadays are minimal."

During the fifteen years after his angiogram in 1980, Rick felt no symptoms of heart trouble. He would go for a stress test once a year and achieved amazing feats on the running machine.

"The only thing was a shortness of breath after about 12 minutes of running fast, and some cramp in the legs. It proved that I was fit. We knew there was a problem, because that would show up on all the systems. The cardiologist would say, jokingly, 'Sooner or later I am going to get you on the operating table.' He was a mad supporter of the football team my players vowed to hate. He promised, 'I'll get you back for all the things you did to us.'"

In March 1996 he was short of breath when walking uphill, although he slept well that night. Next morning at work he went upstairs to his office after a routine inspection of the plant.

"I battled like hell to get up the stairs. I was really having difficulty breathing. Rang the doctor, got into my car and drove home, told him the story, and he was absolutely horrified to think that I'd even drive my car to see him. Made me sit there while he called the cardiologist."

Rick was registered at a private hospital with instructions that his wife was to drive him there immediately. Next day he had an angiogram.

"The decision was made for me on the recommendation of the cardiologist, who I respect and trust. The surgeon, a fine guy, made it all sound so simple. I was going to be in good hands. I had been sedated because I was getting a pain coming up towards my neck. One of the blockages was starting to close off, and they were giving me tablets to make the blood very thin, and try to settle me down. It is very frightening. The cardiologist said, 'I can give you a tablet to take. If you get short of breath, stop for a minute, and you'll be okay. Or we get it right with open-heart surgery. Your car is near here. You may need a tablet by the time you get to it. Knowing you, that's not your lifestyle. So I've arranged for Thursday night open-heart surgery. Five blockages that we want to fix. What do you think? I'll leave you and your wife for a minute.' I looked at my wife, and she indicated it's got to be done. I said to him, 'Don't go. Fine. Thursday night.' He said, 'I've got the surgeon picked out that I want to do it. He's very good, very skilful.'"

(4)

In hospital before the operation

Becoming a patient

If you are an emergency case, events will moved swiftly; if not then you will be eased into the hospital way of life. In either case you will become aware of an important change in your life for a week at least. In this change you will lose much of your everyday control and the feeling of autonomy you normally enjoy, as you are gradually but firmly led into the role of being a patient.

As time goes by, and the technology of hospital life becomes clearer to you, you will be treated as if you were a child. This will not last long, but the feeling of being like a child is sometimes hard to accept. As you get closer to the time of the operation the experience of not being in charge of your life becomes essential to your welfare. This feeling in patients is familiar to the hospital staff, and they make sure that it does not interfere with your welfare by keeping you well informed about what is to take place. In this way, childlike dependence begins to give over to feelings of childlike trust. As confidence re-emerges you return to normal and feel you are an adult again.

People who need a heart bypass operation immediately have no time to prepare for becoming a hospital patient or planning rehabilitation. Others have time to think ahead, consider what to take to hospital, attend to work demands, and plan for their recovery. For those with time, the important items for the hospital are medical certificates, blood type, hospital information, a list of medications, information about health insurance, relevant information on your health problems and your official medical card. You will need some night attire for at least one night before the operation, paper tissues, shoes without laces, underwear, clothes to wear home, and basic toiletries. Women are advised to get themselves a new bra before the operation to limit chest pain from the movement of the breasts after surgery.

Brad was 44 when he had his first operation in January 1980. With time to prepare, he wrote an account of his ill health for his business partners, and rescheduled his work in order to follow the surgeon's directions to prepare for the operation. The hospital took him as soon as it had a place, and recommended until then he should rest.

"They said, 'Don't mow the lawns. Wait, take things quietly.' They recommended against work. I still kept walking, no particular exercises. No heavy gardening. I'd been doing fairly active work, and I relished the thought of reading books I wanted to read rather than books for work."

Two weeks before his operation Lachlan had to stop taking anti-clotting agents for his blood. He took into hospital a small cassette recorder to keep him amused.

"I took in a Walkman with a tape of Garrison Keillor's *Lake Wobegon Days*, and it was absolutely wonderful. I'd be lying in bed laughing my head off. Others couldn't understand why I laughed all the time."

Most hospitals have television and radio available for each patient. You may recover rapidly enough to need your crossword dictionary, writing pad, a list of phone numbers, knitting, sewing or a special book.

You can ask relatives and friends to bring you items you need when they visit with news of the outside world and fresh night attire or underwear.

Arriving at the hospital

When providing hospital office staff with personal information, you will have to say whether or not you have hospital insurance.

In emergencies it does not matter whether or not the patient is insured—the treatment is carried out immediately.

Kim questioned the relevance of hospital insurance, but in retrospect dismissed the financial matters.

"I don't know why they ask that question because the character next to me wasn't insured, and he got operated on by my surgeon, at the same time, and he saved himself a lot of bucks in private fees. Got the same service as I did! Anyway, irrelevant as it goes."

If you are not an emergency patient you will be admitted to hospital in the afternoon, and if you come with a friend or relative they must leave before the day is out. At this point you are under the hospital's control. Liam recalled how he was drawn into the hospital's regime and saw that its routine would soon take over his life for weeks or more.

"They gave me admission sheets and information about what to take to hospital when I went in overnight for the angiogram. Also some commonly asked questions by patients. When I went for bypass surgery they sent me information on the heart and what bypass surgery entailed that I could read lying in bed."

Peter did not like going to hospital, because it limited his personal autonomy, and he resisted the demands to become a pliant and responsive patient for as long as he could.

"I suppose I got there about four. I think they wanted you after lunch and I'd felt there's no way I'm getting there before late afternoon. They *had* wanted me there in the *morning*! I said, 'No, I can't be bothered.' It's because I've got some inkling of hospitals. I detest hospitals, and I thought if I get there I'm just going to hang around while they do what they want to do at *their* pace, if I get there late they'll have to do the bypass. From my point of view *I'm* in control."

Explaining the procedure

Before the operation, many people will see you, and tell you the role they have in your operation and recovery. Explanations vary depending on the different roles medical staff play, what they assume you want to know, and what they think you can understand about medical procedures. With little detail the technical procedures are usually described by your surgeon and anaesthetist, while others offer you an outline of what they think you want to hear.

Erik's surgeon used a model of the heart to show what he would be doing, but he learned little from the anaesthetist.

David was to be operated on very shortly after the medical staff learned how serious his heart disease was. There was no time to say what would be happening, no choices left to him, and one comfort was offered which he did not need.

"A chaplain came in, asked me whether I wanted to discuss anything. I said, 'No. I'm not a religious man.'"

Hank found that once he was in hospital he was made fully aware of what was involved. And, like David, he was approached by a hospital chaplain.

"I watched a film. The surgeon sat down and talked. Others gave you books, and you played with models, and they said, 'This here's blocked, and that too.' Plenty of information about hearts. There were religious people around, but they weren't forcing themselves on you."

Peter had little interest in technical information about his diseased heart and the doctors' procedures. Not competent to appreciate their work, he left everything to them. He arrived for an operation like a customer coming to a shop.

"My view was, 'I'm not conscious, you're in charge, I assume you're competent. Do the job. That's it.' I can't recall being prepared for the operation ... The surgeon popped in. Nurses and the anaesthetist popped in and he said, 'Hello, I'm your anaesthetist.' He may've indicated what he would do, but I wasn't terribly interested."

In Brad's case it was the physiotherapist and the anaesthetist who explained the procedure for his first bypass operation.

"I had a fair idea as to what going to happen and it didn't overly worry me. The anaesthetist mentioned the uncomfortable respirator tube down your throat. I was ready for it. That helped."

At the hospital on the evening before the operation, the surgeon came to see Chris and took him through the procedure in detail.

"I felt he would have preferred those days when a surgeon didn't have to meet you or explain anything at all ... He asked, 'Happy for me to go ahead?' I said, 'Of course, otherwise I'll drop dead.'"

Not long before the operation the staff insisted, against his wishes, that Chris watch a video of a the surgical procedure itself, and an anaesthetist came in for a few minutes to see if he was allergic to any medication that might be used during the operation.

"He asked if I was allergic to anything. I told him one thing commonly used in surgery. The previous time that I'd had it I had been violently ill for days. He noted that and disappeared."

Barbara learned from acquaintances who had undergone the operation that the cut would be down through her sternum, and that her body would be chilled. Her surgeon confirmed those details and using a sketch showed there would be three bypasses. James also learned much about the operation from people whom he knew personally. Otherwise he was informed at the hospital.

Lachlan learned something of the medical procedure, and recalled that valuable information on problems of recovery had come from the man who shaved him before the operation. More details of the technical procedure would not have been welcome.

"They said that you'll be put on a heart–lung machine to keep your blood oxygenated so nothing's going to happen to your vital functions. But they didn't tell you that your heart was actually stopped, or how the machine operated while you're unconscious, or about the recovery, or the risks of this operation. The surgeon said this is the operation, and that it was not *perfectly* safe, and made reference to non-clotting procedures. But the man who shaved me said, 'After the operation you're going to need to cough ... because your lungs will be full of gunk.' That was the level of the explanation. I didn't know anything of the procedures. There wasn't any need, and it's traumatic if you think about it."

A doctor checked Catherine each day while she waited for a vacancy at the hospital where her operation would be done.

He described the blockages around her heart. At the hospital her family were with her when the anaesthetist explained the procedure.

On the night before the operation Rick saw his surgeon and anaesthetist and a medical team prepared his body for surgery. He was told not to hesitate about asking anyone any question at all.

Giving consent

Your surgeon cannot operate without your legal consent. When you become a patient for heart bypass surgery you will be expected to sign a form. By signing this form you give your informed consent to the operation, agreeing that you know what the operation is for, and that you want the named surgeon to perform the procedure.

Most people find the document is too difficult to follow because it is cast in unfamiliar legal terms. A lawyer can help you with this. The document assumes that you trust the surgeon, regard them as most competent, and believe the medical staff will do their best should some unexpected complication occur. The form also implies that you understand the risk of serious surgery, and problems that might follow. If you feel anxious about what you are signing, talk with the surgeon.

In hindsight the document has many meanings. Kim and Erik saw the document as a legal move to prevent them from suing the medical staff should something go wrong.

Hank signed something—he could not remember what—and Chris remembered vaguely that he too had signed something but could not recall who had given it to him. Ethan, James and Barbara had similar memories, and Catherine said she recalled that it did not matter much to her at the time.

But signing *did* matter to Peter, because it meant a further loss of autonomy in his becoming a patient.

> "I'm sure I signed something, somewhere, but I couldn't honestly tell you what or how or when. I didn't go through it line by line. I was told I needed a bypass, I believed them, therefore let them get on with it. I had infinite faith in it. There's nothing you can do."

Liam was the only informant who remembered that the anaesthetist was as involved as the surgeon in requiring informed consent.

"Informed consent was done that afternoon with two consent forms, one for surgery and one for the anaesthetic, presented by the nurse who was looking after me. She said, 'Of course, you know for us to do this you need to agree to consent to these procedures.' Just a *pro forma*. Both of them half a page."

Visiting the intensive care ward

Today more patients are shown what they look like when they come from the operating room to be cared for in the hospital's intensive care unit (ICU). In the past it was thought unnecessary and probably too frightening to show the patient to those in the ICU. You are not a pretty sight.

Not all informants saw patients in Intensive Care, and not all wanted to see them. If you are given the opportunity, you do not have to go to the ICU. Perhaps it would be better for your relatives to see others in Intensive Care so that they would know how you would look after the operation.

Erik was assured that in Intensive Care he would look a mess of tubes and monitors. But he himself was glad to know that his wife would be prepared for the sight of him.

"What I liked was on the day *before* the operation they asked her to come into the intensive care ward so that she wouldn't be frightened when she saw me, a horrific sight. People with tubes sticking out all over the place can be a frightening experience. It's a good idea to take the patient down there, and say, 'That's what you look like, but you'll be all right. So don't get a fright.'"

Two days before his operation Rick saw the intensive care unit, but Hank and Tanner were not taken there, nor was David. This bothered David because when his daughter saw him after the operation she cried. Barbara was supposed to be shown the intensive care unit, but she had deteriorated so much that she was put on a drip and could not be moved. She was pleased to learn that her husband had been there.

"My husband went down and saw it, and talked to other patients. That was a comfort. I didn't want to see it or bother opening my eyes. That was my way of coping with it."

Liam visited the ICU and learned much about the place without entering the unit itself. The visit did not distress him but reassured him about events immediately after the operation.

> "I could see how the twelve beds were arranged, with a central monitoring point. Monitors were above the beds, each patient having their individual nurse all the time on a twelve-hour shift. And the doctor doing a twelve-hour shift. I glimpsed the patients in a fully active ICU. He said, 'One of those spots is going to be you in about twelve hours' time.'"

Physical preparation for the operation

After learning about the procedure, you are then prepared physically for the operation: with blood tests, X-rays, cleaning your body, and ensuring that your stomach is empty.

In the evening before the operation you shower with a special antiseptic soap, and next day you take another shower, or may be bathed by a nurse. This makes sure that you are free of anything that might harbour infection or unacceptable bacteria. Erik recalled the experience.

> "You've got to shower yourself in the evening before you go back to bed and again in the morning when you get up. They supply you with antiseptic soap. A guy came with an electric shaver. All over your body, your legs especially, and your groin, and your chest obviously. When they wake you, you shower again and they give you a gown. You don't put your pyjamas on again. They come and wheel you in."

Hank had a lot of body hair, so he was shaved the day before the operation. Chris, Brad, and David also remembered being shaved shortly before the operation, but Barbara was too unwell to remember details of the preparation. Her health had declined rapidly and she needed her operation sooner than anticipated.

As part of his preparation, after being shaved, James's legs were marked for the removal of his saphenous vein.

> "You're shaved all over your chest, and legs because they take the vein out of the leg. They look at the veins and mark the veins of your leg with a blue stain."

Unlike James, Peter was able to indicate which of the leg veins was to be removed.

"They wanted to shave both my legs, and I said, 'No way you're going to shave *both* legs. You'll have to take the vein you want from that leg because that leg's been cut open once before in another operation. So you can't do that.' So we decided to do that, because if it wasn't shaved they wouldn't cut it."

Liam was to be operated on at eight in the morning, so his preparation had to begin early. The nurse warned him the night before that preparation would begin at five next morning, and that she would be waking him up.

Nil orally

Most informants were told not to eat for 8 to 10 hours before the operation. Erik, David, and Chris stopped eating after a meal the night before their operation, while Catherine was mistakenly offered breakfast on the morning of her operation:

"That morning I was not to have breakfast. A breakfast tray was presented to me and I laughed, and I said, 'You've made a mistake. Please take it away.'"

Liam was to have his operation early in the morning, and from the nurse learned why it was necessary to cease eating so long beforehand. This was followed by a session with the dietician.

"First, the general nurse said, 'You're down for 8 o'clock in the morning, so you're nil orally because of the food being thrown back up if you have a seizure. We'll give you fluids until about 10 o'clock tonight.'"

From the dietician Liam learned that in fact he would *not* be interested in food after the operation, that his eating would change, and he would follow a new eating regimen for the rest of his life.

"Second, a dietitian said, 'You won't be eating for a few days, but I want to check your usual diet, to see how we can change it so your new pipes don't clog up the way the other ones did.' She was treating heart disease as an entity, talking about different types of cholesterol. She started preventative education at that stage."

Having the operation

Having the operation delayed or brought forward

At the last minute, operations can be put off or brought forward. Emergencies may arise, and your operation could be delayed for several hours while a more urgent case is dealt with; or perhaps your own health may decline so rapidly that you are put up higher on the list. Catherine was delayed for over a week, Erik for a few hours; Kim was delayed a week because he was ill, while Barbara became an emergency and was first off the rank for that day.

> "They moved me up to the top of the list when it was clear I was going downhill. First off the rank. I had been told I was second or third. By morning they had me number one."

The operation itself

Heart bypass patients recall nothing about the operation itself. The last images you see involve hazy feelings about being moved from room to room, lights, voices of medical staff, a little banter, a feeling that instructions are being given, and occasional questions being put until you are asleep. Only the medical staff know the details of the operation.

Among the medical staff are the chief surgeon and usually two assistants, three nurses, two anaesthetists, a technician to operate the heart–lung machine, and an electronic engineer to maintain the equipment. Much preparation is needed before the operation itself, so you are brought, sedated, to the operating room about two hours beforehand.

Details of the procedure can be read in medical books, and seen either on videos available to medical students in medical libraries or in atlases on heart surgery. As Hank put it, 'You wouldn't want to know about it.' From the surgeon's point of view the operation can be exhausting; it is long, requires intense concentration, close attention to detail, and carries the responsibilities and anxieties of exercising full authority over a life and death procedure.

What follows is a non-technical summary of the main events during the heart bypass operation. The events vary with the surgeon, the patient, the number of arteries needing attention, and the hospital organisation of its resources. As more becomes known about heart disease, and the technical procedures are refined and extended, the description of a heart bypass operation becomes more out of date.

As a rule, work begins with an anaesthetist giving different intravenous infusions, and attaching you to a monitoring system for the duration of the operation. The surgical work itself will take about five hours, depending on the patient.

At first a vein is removed from your leg, maybe both legs, or from your forearm. It will be used to replace the blood vessel at the point around your heart where the free flow of blood is blocked. You are cut from the base of the neck to the abdomen, and then, using an electric saw, your surgeon cuts down the centre of your chest bone, the sternum, and your rib cage is opened to the right and left and secured in place with a spreader.

Your heart is in view. The surgeon removes a mammary artery that runs down the back of the breastbone, clamps it to stop the bleeding and puts it aside. After opening the sac around your heart, the pericardium, the surgeon connects your heart and lung system to a heart–lung bypass machine, variously known as a 'pump' or a 'washing machine'. Your heart is stopped and chilled. You are now literally having your 'bypass'.

Most open-heart surgery requires the pump to circulate nourishing blood to the body while the heart has been stopped. During this preparation for heart surgery the major blood vessels are connected to the machine.

Using high-powered magnifying glasses, the surgeon sews the harvested blood vessel to the blocked coronary artery. The thread is strong and as fine as human hair. This grafted blood vessel will carry your blood around the point where once it had been blocked. In most operations, three blocked points can be bypassed this way—a triple bypass.

Your heart is then started with an electric charge and is filled with warm blood. The heart–lung bypass machine is turned off, and, as your lungs revive, the repaired heart begins to work again. Once this is established, the breastbone is drawn back over your heart and lungs and stapled together at the centre, and your leg wounds are sewn up. To inflate your lungs a respirator tube is put down your throat into your windpipe. This uncomfortable tube passes between your vocal cords, so you cannot speak until it has done its work and been taken out.

Thin wires can be seen coming out of the base of your chest, and tubes are also placed there to drain unwanted blood from around the heart. Other tubes may be used to help empty your bladder and stomach. Fluids are given to you through narrow intravenous tubes in the neck, arms or legs. When you are first seen by friends and relations you look a mess of wires and tubes.

The natural fear of death

In general, the risk of dying during the operation is between one and three per cent, and the risk of a heart attack during the operation is about five per cent. However slim the statistical chances of dying are, the subjective risk for each person is felt deeply and uniquely, but managed differently.

Liam and Catherine accepted the anticipation of death as a natural fear, but coped in their own way. In hospital on the night before the operation, Liam attempted to put thoughts of death aside without much success; he was offered a sedative to help him sleep that night, but refused on principle. Thinking little could be achieved by his wife's staying with him, he sent her home, but still wanted to have someone with him to talk. This led to his debating whether or not it would have been better to have been put into a room with others rather than a private ward.

"My wife stayed until about 6 o'clock and then I said, 'Look, nothing's achieved by hanging around, go home.' Through the night I had a fair amount of anxiety and the nurse asked, 'Do you want to take a tranquilliser or something?' Probably I should've, but I thought, 'To hell with it!' Couldn't read, couldn't concentrate. I was listening to music, which was helpful. I'm in two minds whether I should've been in a larger ward with others. I don't know. I couldn't really focus. I didn't want the effort of talking to others, and yet it might've been better. A natural fear would come and go while I was lying around waiting in preparation, and during the two or three weeks before going into hospital. Without telling my wife I drew up a will. It *was* scary. I'm not heroic. About one o'clock I got to sleep."

Catherine controlled her fear of death by not thinking that it affected her until after the operation, by attributing such fear to others in her family, and by recalling that she had kept death at bay for so many years.

"Over the years it didn't really worry me because it had always been controlled. It didn't seem to affect me in any great way. My family worried more than I did. I had been very active, and here I was hospitalised. I wasn't afraid until it was all over and done with."

Lachlan accepted the operation, and, on balance, the risk of dying, and turned the anxiety about death onto his wife, and the explanation for his illness onto his occupation.

"I knew that I might not come round, but if I didn't have the operation I wouldn't be walking round anyway. I was rather sanguine about it all. My wife was more worried than me when a health regime was laid down. I was 53—a common age for men to have heart attacks. So I didn't worry about it."

Like Catherine and Lachlan, David not only denied fear of death and attributed to others, but also controlled it by placing the dark side of the operation in the hands of others.

"I didn't have any fear of not coming back. I feel sure my wife did, and I feel sure the kids did. But I had absolutely no fear about it all. Someone told me it had to be done—so it had to be done. I was more than happy because I knew my father had died from it."

Hank accepted the inevitable, and his fear was that if he didn't have the operation, he would explode in death. After the operation he was comforted by his wife's belief that death had been put aside, thus making his fear irrelevant.

> "It was pretty scary. I had a time bomb ticking away in my chest. It was a matter of time before it went off. It *had* gone off, and someone was looking after me, like God, or whatever. Then I was in the right place at the right time and the right things happened. I ended up going through the system and being fixed. Afterwards my wife kept saying, 'Don't worry, you've been fixed, there's nothing to worry about.'"

Death became irrelevant in Chris's approach to the operation when he said, 'If I don't have surgery I'm going to die anyway, so what does it matter?'

Death was not irrelevant to Kim; it returned—and was banished again—when he was asked to sign the informed consent document.

> "I'm not scared of death whatsoever. More Scorpios commit suicide than any other star sign, worldwide. The only scary thing you have is when they get you to sign a paper saying that you may die, and that's a reminder that this might kill me."

To Peter the operation was inevitable. He did not want to listen to the evidence that death might be near, nor dwell on the risks of the procedure, so he compared the operation he was about to have with a successful operation on his back almost forty years ago.

Feelings before operation

The night before the operation the patient's mind fills with private imaginings, hope and anxiety. But what can be done in those last twenty-four hours? Catherine felt a 'reassuring feeling most of the time' because 'everything had been taken care of'. Erik was confident of his surgeon and about the future, no matter which way things turned out.

> "I felt so confident the night before the operation, I slept like a baby. I had the attitude—it might sound ridiculous now—but I know I did: I'm not 35, right? I didn't miss out on anything in life; and I was so confident in the surgeon. I was so utterly confident that I felt, 'If I wake up I will be all right. If I don't wake up I'm no worse off either.'"

An uncomfortable tube down his throat was the main thought occupying Peter.

"I only have one fear of operations. With hay fever my throat gets pretty damn raw, and that thing they stick down your throat frightens me because I feel I'm going to choke, gag on it."

Lachlan felt he was a healthy man of 53, no diabetes, did not smoke, and, apart from having an inadequate supply of blood to the heart, was in relatively good health. The hospital was free of most diseases. And what could he want?

"If the operation's going to occur, and you've said to somebody to organise it, then it's organised."

Comfort from others at the hospital

Heart surgery stirs deep feelings about oneself. Family and friends share the feelings, and others may call to wish good luck. David felt comforted by a friend's advice that the operation was easy to recover from, Chris enjoyed yarning with the hospital chaplain about dignitaries in the church, and Barbara felt greatly supported by the realistic views of both the chaplain and the nurses who gave time to talk with her.

"The nurses talked about it, and did not pretend it wasn't going to be traumatic. I asked to see the chaplain. He had had the operation, which was very helpful. And he was quite open about it, not dramatic, but he pointed out that it would be very painful, which nobody else had ever said."

Going into the operation

After being prepared physically for the operation, you are made as calm as possible. Gradually you become aware that you no longer control your future and must not do anything but lie still and go with the flow of the medical procedure. This state of mind is achieved with various drugs that relax your muscles, help you feel comfortable, and promote a sense of well-being, even light-heartedness. However doped or woozy you feel, there are some traces of your going into the operation that stay with you because you are not utterly unconscious; some images persist and maintain clarity, while others become vague and defy memory. Lasting images appear to be related to interruptions in the flow of uncontrollable events.

Under effective sedation Liam, Lachlan, David, and Chris seem to have been ideal patients going into an operation. Liam and Lachlan recalled the moments before unconsciousness in much detail; David remembered very little.

Liam seemed to become part of the technical procedure he had expected.

"The nurse washes me ... I have a sip of water. I'm not groggy, but the Valium is having an effect, and I'm quite perky. The gown is done up at the back while you are in bed and then they come for you with a special trolley ... I am quite relaxed, not much emotion at all. I feel, 'Okay! Let's get on with it.' No feeling of resignation. Bit more *gung ho* than that. They wheel you ... up to the operating room on the next floor where all the medical gang are, their fancy masks on and saying cheerfully, 'Hello! Well, here you are. You probably can't recognise me behind the mask.' ... Surgeon says, 'Well, I suppose we might as well get on with it' ... Anaesthetist says, 'Okay, and this is where you count backwards.' I say, 'Yeah, I've been expecting that.' And something goes into the back of my hand, I count back from ten, nine, here we are, this is it."

Lachlan also oriented himself to this half-conscious world. He was surprised to learn his anaesthetist had an assistant, and remembered having a drug to quieten him down while being moved off, feeling dopey, and surrounded by a hazy impression that the organisation behind the operation was sending him through several interconnected rooms filled with sounds of medical staff at work, issuing instructions and talking to each other. With each move he felt more settled.

"I remember the catheter going into the back of my hand and I am not at all fussed ... I remember a bell being rung, the door is opened ... I am being wheeled into an intermediate area, like going through an air lock ... Into a room. Are the lights on, or is it *really* dim? They are talking, but I can't remember what they are saying. They pat your hand and say, 'How are you doing?' Between the two anaesthetists ... I vaguely remember instructions are being passed ... I have the feeling that the two nurses are talking about what they'd been doing at the weekend."

Like Lachlan and Liam, Brad recalled the medical staff talking moments before he was unconscious, notably the anaesthetist, who kept Brad informed of what was happening.

"The pre-med was given, an injection or a tablet. I have on the usual hospital gown, and I am waiting in a preparing room. In the operating people are talking, but I don't see the surgeon then. The anaesthetist has told me very little beforehand. Whether that's a good or a bad thing I'm not too sure. But now he says, 'I'll now give you a little prick in the wrist.' He kept me informed as he went along."

Hank, Barbara, and Catherine had anxious moments during the final stage of preparation. Hank managed by talking himself into a relaxed state, and was then taken further with the drugs.

"In the pre-op room I am pretty nervous. I am saying, 'You're fit, you're young, they do this to *old* people. *You've* got nothing to worry about.' I think everybody is nervous. It's a big day. They give me something, take me down to the room beside the operating room and give me something there. They knock you out in stages, and get you nice and relaxed."

Shortly before the operation, a nurse seemed unable to assess Barbara's blood sugar level. Distressed by what appeared to be incompetence, Barbara lost trust in the nurse. Later she concluded that probably her own emotions affected the blood sugar reading more than usual.

"Before the operation a nurse came up with a horrendously low blood sugar reading for me, and I said, 'I don't think that's right.' 'Oh, yes,' she replied. But I believed that if I'd been as low as *that* I would barely have been *conscious*. I went round to the nurses' station and said, 'I wish to have my blood sugar tested again.' They rang my specialist, and he said, 'Don't do anything.' If he had said, as he could've, 'Give her extra insulin,' I would have passed out in the night! My next reading was normal. Emotions can make a big difference with your sugar reading. In the operating room they talked to me, but I was too relaxed to remember anything else."

Early in the morning Catherine was lonely, and felt keen to get the operation over with. Drugs calmed her, and, like others, she found comfort from the talk in the operating room.

"Early I felt alone. I didn't need anything. I didn't see anyone. So I took myself to a recreation room and I tried to read. Wasn't interested. One o'clock for my surgery, but then it was made later in the day. So I had a long time without food. Some pre-op medication was delivered into the back of my hand. I am becoming fidgety, I want get it over and done with, so I can start getting better. The pre-op injections calm me, and finally I am taken to the operation and hear interesting conversations going on around me. I am partly in the conversation because some of it is about me. I feel included, and they are not talking over my head. I am just lying there, being discussed."

Peter was anxious too, but he had a friendly, detached attitude to the anaesthetist. This helped him manage his concern about the operation by putting all responsibility into the hands of the medical staff, and, unlike Catherine, he felt he was not part of the group at the operation; instead, he enjoyed the early stages of his unconsciousness:

"I always find that little trip on the trolley where you're passing out is the most delightful experience."

Rick had the comfort of knowing that he was feeling cheerful about the operation, and made one last attempt to be sure his wife would do what he wanted while others were wheeling him away from her.

"The injections were being given to me, and tablets to keep me down. I became very drowsy in the afternoon, and then my wife said I became hyped up, saying funny things, joking, being smart. She said, 'When you were wheeled off, you were on a high.' I remember saying, 'Don't you move from there. I'll be back!'"

6

In Intensive Care

During the operation, your body will have undergone devastating trauma, and been shocked into a state very close to death. After the operation the first stage of recovery is in a surgical intensive care unit (SICU or ICU). You have a respirator tube down your windpipe past the vocal cords. It is impossible to speak. Another tube empties your bladder and there is another for the stomach. Around the heart are more tubes to drain away accumulated blood and into neck, legs and arms are more tubes to administer drugs and various other fluids. Your blood pressure and the electrical activities of your body are monitored. Wires will have been attached to your heart so that the physician can control your heart rate if necessary.

All your vital functions are closely watched and for most of the time in the intensive care unit you are aware of very little. Some patients are there for a half a day, others for two days. When you are well enough, much of the equipment will be removed, and you will be moved to a ward nearby where you are monitored closely until it is clear you are ready to go to a ward, or a room of your own. The time spent at each stage of intensive care is a technical decision taken by the medical staff.

It is difficult to understand the organisation surrounding the operation and your time in intensive care afterwards. You are drifting in and out of consciousness and are aware of stages in the organised recovery, which may be held up for many reasons, especially if the heart rate is too high or low. On one hand you may feel so bad that you do not want anyone to see you like this; on the other, you may appreciate the opportunity to dream strange things.

Most informants felt pleased to be the centre of attention, and even surprised at how well they had managed the operation, and that they were lucky, and had started getting better. Probably the only thing that can be done to help the recovery at this stage is to warn family and friends that you will not look yourself for at least twenty-four hours, and they should not be too concerned, anxious or angry to see you helpless, physically distorted, and unable to say to them how you feel. Things can only get better.

Your inner life will tell you not only about some unconscious world of self-distortions, hallucinations, and time loss, but also the pleasant discovery that after having been so near death you are actually alive.

Because the pain is unbearable, drugs are used to help you cope. But you can become addicted to the drugs because they work so well in relieving pain and for some people help produce happy hallucinations and dreams. You might feel your breathing tighten, and feel the pain return when you believed it was going; however, you will appreciate the nurse who helped prevent you from becoming a drug addict, and you will find ways to manage the pain by positioning your body to get relief, and by comparing your current pain with earlier experiences. In a small way, you are beginning to increase control over your recovery.

Your appearance to others after your operation

If your family and friends have not been to see patients in the intensive care unit, they will probably be shocked at the sight of your body, and how drained you feel and how helpless you appear. James's wife said the sight of him gave her an incredible fright, and the elaborate technology reminded her of something from outer space; this sight surprised and distressed David's daughter when she came to see him. She had researched many aspects of medicine, and he thought she would be more familiar with what had been done with him immediately after the operation.

"She knew all these things, except the shock of walking in and seeing me like that. Tubes everywhere. She cried to see her dad like that. My wife was all right. Other family members were good."

Hank's family were not only shocked, but also distressed by the long daily journey to the city and back home to see him.

"All the family visited me in hospital. They were shocked at what had happened. I was at the city hospital for fourteen days. The whole thing took a month from the heart attack day until the day I came home. I was quite a drain on the immediate family, as they had to go up to the city so often."

Brad's parents also lived out of town, and his own family were relieved that they were unable to come to the city to see their son in such a state after the operation.

"I think they were all a bit shocked by how I looked and they said it was just as well my parents, being pretty old then, hadn't come to the hospital from their country town. They would've been a bit shocked. It's not a pretty sight. I mean when you look at the other guys round you, with this thing in your mouth and with tubes everywhere. It looks worse than it is, probably. In fact it's not a bad operation painwise at all compared with others."

Chris recalled that it was the shape of his limbs that shocked his family.

"The nurses told me afterwards that the family goes into a terrible shock when they see you. I was only wearing something across my middle. Just a towel or something. Apparently my whole body—particularly my fingers and toes—were all swollen. Looked like minute sausages. That gave them a fright. They were assured that this was quite normal. There was nothing strange about it."

Coming to

Immediately after the operation, most informants drifted in and out of consciousness, unable to recall exactly what was happening, where they were, or how long they spent in Intensive Care. They learned about that from others.

Liam's wife visited him in Intensive Care after a call from the surgeon.

"I really was *non compos mentis* in ICU, just coming in and out. I made some eye contact with the nurse who was looking after me, and the surgeon —smiles and waves. I was pretty much bombed out during those two days.

The kids came in and a close friend. Didn't really talk much. No food, only a bit of orange juice. After ICU there's what they called a 'post-cardiac' or 'thoracic' unit, it's a transition ward, with further monitoring but not so intense as ICU."

Catherine's heart was 'racing' so she stayed in Intensive Care a little longer than she thought was normal, and felt she had became the centre of attention. This gave her time to observe what was going on, to recall the distress of not being allowed to drink.

"I was in there for two and a half days instead of one and a half days because the heart rate was racing ... I was fascinated with the fact that I was connected up to a computer. Even my blinking was registered, and there were people sitting there noting all these things. I wasn't eating, but I was dreadfully thirsty and I wasn't allowed to drink. I was allowed to have ice-cubes and a face washer. I remember that dreadful thirst."

Peter relied on his wife for his knowledge of life in the Intensive Care unit. After a day in the ICU he was put into a room nearby and was closely monitored.

"The intensive care room—I really have no memory whatsoever. I was 24 hours in intensive care, two days in the monitoring room, and then put into the private room. My wife says I was only three or four hours in intensive care. I can remember coming to, and this damn thing was in my throat, and felt I was going to choke. They put the pethidine in and I passed out again."

Erik was in Intensive Care for the best part of two days, had nothing to drink, but recalled that a nurse may have wet his mouth occasionally, and that he was not fed. David believed that he was in intensive care for six to ten hours, or perhaps a day, before being taken to a ward.

Hank was not sure how long his operation lasted or how long he was in intensive care, but recalls that on the day after the operation there were plans to have him taken to a ward. But he seemed to be aware of who was there in the intensive care unit.

"I'm not sure how long I was in the ICU. They did me on a Monday, and by Tuesday they were wanting to get me into an ordinary ward. I'm not sure how long the operation lasted. When you wake up in ICU there is someone there ... I had no family or friends there, but other people had their people with them. I think my wife was there when I made it back to the room."

Waking up in discomfort

After coming to, waking in Intensive Care is both joyous and unpleasant. You are alive and will be feeling better, but down your throat you have an uncomfortable endotracheal breathing tube to help your deflated lungs clear and function effectively again. Few people recall painful details of waking because, it seems, time diminishes the discomfort and heals the pain, and other memories find ways to dominate your recovery.

On his way to the operation room Rick had ordered his wife not to leave, he'd be back. But it didn't work out like that.

"I woke up in a small room, lights and people moving, things banging. I wondered where the hell I was. I couldn't move because my arms were pinned to my side and I had this terrible thing in my mouth. I didn't know this would be in my mouth, or that my arms would be pinned to my side."

Hank was also greatly affected by the tube down his throat, and strangely sensitive to the unpleasant noise of a nurse walking around.

"I came out quickly, and can remember being totally aggravated by a nurse walking with squeaky shoes. Quite angry. I've vivid memories of gagging, a terrifying, horrible experience. Like I was drowning in my own phlegm. This tube is down your throat, and it's doing your breathing for you. Apparently a lot of people don't even know about it. Until they got this thing out I thought that I was going to choke fighting this thing."

Watched by his wife and daughter, Chris woke in Intensive Care. People came and went. He could see other patients hooked up to equipment. He had a drip but no memory of anything else, until it came time to eat!

"I was suddenly aware of two people at the end of the bed ... I was breathing, and there were people talking to me. I couldn't talk because I had a tube down my throat. All that would come out was 'Ugh'. This gave me a surprise. I wanted to say, 'Why the hell is my throat so sore? Everything feels so thick.' So the nurse pulled over a blackboard. My wife asked, 'What do you feel like?' I wrote, 'I want to eat.' 'What do you want to eat?' I wrote, 'Two dozen oysters!' With this thing in my throat I imagined an oyster, cool and refreshing, sliding down my throat."

David remembered some details of waking up and was surprised that he did not feel ill, although he was shocked by the tube down his throat. Upset by his daughter's distress and unable to speak, he wrote in big letters on the bedspread the promise he had made to his family.

"They should have told me beforehand that I would have a thing blocking my throat. That was a big shock. You couldn't see or move. Tubes were all coming out of the lower chest and out of my neck. But they were fantastic people in that recovery centre; they watched me. I watched the doctor who happened to be this absolutely beautiful Asian girl. I thought I was in paradise! At the other end of the bed was a fantastic male nurse. He put water over my tube to wet my mouth. My daughter was there, crying to see her dad like that. I couldn't talk. On the bed cover I wrote T-U-S-C-A-N-Y. My wife wanted to go to Tuscany. When I wrote it they all started crying."

Liam woke feeling bruised, in little pain, and with his chest under pressure. His wakening had a joyful tone. Then came a friendly face, an array of tubes rampant, some drug-assisted dreams, and finally a conscious interest focused on the narrow tube in his throat.

"I'm feeling surprised. Between my feet I see the supervising physician. He gives a smile and a wave as he goes by. Very reassuring to see a friendly face. I feel I'm in good hands. Floating in and out of consciousness, beautiful dreams. I can really understand how people get hooked on heroin. Cloud Nine! ... They say when they are going to take the tube out; you put your head back, out it comes. Fantastic relief. I had a very dry throat, and the male nurse held up a cup with the angled straw, nectar, gorgeously cool, sweet flavoured orange juice. One of the high notes of being in ICU is sipping that orange juice."

Although Erik recalled the tube in his throat, he was not interested in pain, but in being alive, and the curious experience of speaking in a familiar language that he believed he had lost.

"You don't wake up. It's like a dream. I said to my wife, 'I'm here.' That was that! I had a pipe in my nose, but I wasn't uncomfortable. My wife told me later that when they bent over the bed I talked in a fluent German that I don't speak any more. My German now is so bad. The moment the nurse came I spoke English, and I did all that with the subconscious."

Brad woke in Intensive Care to hear a nurse's reassuring use of his given name as she helped him to adjust the tube down his throat.

"I heard my name being used, and thought at the time that it's a cunning method to get your attention. Nurse was saying what she was doing and keeping me in touch. I had the thing in the mouth. You tend to fall asleep and forget to breathe. She was saying, 'Now don't fall asleep! Come on, keep breathing.' So you start breathing again. The quicker you did that, the quicker you got this tube out."

James and Barbara recalled nothing of the discomfort in their throat, but Lachlan did. He also imagined a loss of time, the distortion of his appearance by the operation, and a dream that he thought might have been the result of the anaesthetic or painkillers used afterwards. He related much of this to near-death experiences that had affected him earlier.

"I must've been reacting to the dream-inducing morphine. I had hallucinatory experiences … Also I didn't realise what the state of your face is after eight and a half hours of surgery. It is about twice as big as normally … When I had the respirator tube taken out, and was breathing under my own steam, very shallowly, my wife held my hand."

Pain after the operation

After struggling into consciousness, the next task is to manage the unrelenting pain of the surgery; drugs will kill that pain for a few hours, but at the price of an addictive pleasure. At first Liam found the pain unbearable and, like a drug addict, he longed for the painkiller; at the same time his nurse was gradually weaning him from it.

"When you are brought into the monitoring ward they give you a syrup of pain-killer every four hours. Next day, one every six hours. I remember by the fourth hour you were in strife! It was part of the weaning process, the cold turkey effect. You got nothing for another four hours, and you would last only about three hours, and in that fourth hour—oh, the pain in the chest. Like you hit your shin bone all the way up the shin. You learn not to move too quickly. By the fourth hour you are just looking forward to that red morphine thing like a real junky, you gulp it down and it works within ten minutes. By the fourth day you're onto codeine."

Hank, a fit man in his forties, felt that he had been hit badly. The pain did not go for over a year.

> "It felt as if I'd been hit by a truck … Immediately after the operation you get these strange pains in your chest. I remember talking to an old fellow at the local jetty, and he said, 'Your organs have been sitting there for forty-five years. All of sudden they pull them out and stick them back in. Don't expect there to be no pain at all.' The pain lasted on and off for twelve months, even longer."

Catherine and Brad both had pain in the chest and leg. Chris had heard that some people find the pain in the leg more unbearable than the chest pain. Not so in his case. When the pain-killers were taken away his pain returned.

> "Once they started taking me off pain-killers, the pain in the chest increased, dramatically, a vertical pain right around the cut. I could feel the stainless steel gizmos they'd done me up with inside … Breathing felt tight, arm and shoulder movements were restricted by the drips that I had. As soon as I moved an arm, a drip would pop out. I felt very round-shouldered, which I think was my attempt to minimise the pain by hugging myself."

Like Chris, James did not feel pain to any degree until after a few days the drugs were no longer available.

> "In Intensive Care you're pretty well drugged so you don't feel very much at all. No pain at that stage. The pain comes a couple of days later when they take you off the heavy sedation, and they try and make you get out of bed. You think you're going to fall apart. The pain's incredible."

7

Complications after the operation

After the operation most patients recover without trouble; but for a few there are minor inconveniences, for others a few months of unpleasantness, and in some cases long, serious complications. Lasting discomfort and problems are described in chapter 12.

Among the participants, minor complications centred on problems of blood supply, difficulties in breathing, unexpected pain in the shoulder and the foot, and in Kim's case a near-death experience.

Complications in hospital

In the evening after her operation, Barbara believed she was still in Intensive Care, floating in and out of consciousness, when she heard a nurse say that she appeared to be losing blood.

> "The nurse called, 'She's losing more blood than I can put in! Call the surgeon! Call the husband.' I was whizzed back to the operating room, and in the lift I lost consciousness. When I came back from this second time in surgery I had the respirator tube in again. What happened was, when they had cut the sternum ... they sealed it with paste on the inside, and there was a gap in the paste. It hadn't sealed properly and blood was oozing from behind it. Didn't really set me back."

Chris also had two serious but easily managed complications. The first occurred at the end of the operation and made it necessary to start again.

"They *performed* the operation as planned. Double bypass. Used a section of an artery from the chest. Took two to three hours. But the surgery didn't *go* as planned. The artery burst. Real emergency! Blood flowing all over, and a rapidly falling blood pressure. Only thing they could do was take a long section of the vein from the inside of my right leg, and do the whole operation again. I was in the operation for eight to nine hours. I didn't become aware of this until I was in my room a couple of days later. The surgeon explained what had gone wrong. I can't remember exactly what was said. I got such a shock I just turned off. I accepted the fact they had done a repeat and it worked. Otherwise I'd be in the hospital mortuary."

He was aware of the second difficulty, an unexpected blood problem, which arose not long after he was taken back to his room. Later Chris learned that he had had a violent and rare reaction to a certain blood type. The blood had been tested thoroughly, and his reaction was totally unexpected. With the anaemia problem solved he was given tablets and the pain and related difficulties vanished.

James had two serious problems in hospital. The first he was not aware of, and the second he recalled, but without distress. After the operation he learned that he too had bled profusely, and that there was talk of reopening him, but it was not necessary. Later he felt his heart start to behave extraordinarily, and this worried him. His breathing was impaired by a lung collapse, not an unusual problem.

"I wasn't aware until many days later that I did bleed a lot after the operation and they were considering reopening me. But because I was young, only 50, they left it, and it was all right. But later in the ward my heart went berserk, the machine freaked out, and I was terrified it wouldn't work! The doctor said that I had an irritable heart, it's been disturbed and will just settle down. It did. On the third day I did breathing exercises and one of my lungs had collapsed—reasonably common, I believe—and that was one of the reasons I was tired. The physiotherapist suggested that I go to the classes for rehabilitation after I came home, which I did."

Brad, too, had difficulty with breathing after the operation, and also had valuable advice from his physiotherapist at the hospital.

"I had a semi-collapse or a collapse of the left lung, and they worked on that. It was a surprise to them. I knew I'd be getting physio to help me breathe deeply, and she told me why. She was so good. I got more information out of that one person than I did out of any other."

In Intensive Care, Rick had an unusual pain, and frustrated, found he could not tell anyone about it.

"The most enormous, horrendous pain in my left shoulder. But I couldn't tell anybody because of the thing in my mouth, and because my hands were kept down at my sides They knew that there was something wrong. In and out of unconsciousness, and this blasted pain was still there. Eventually, they took this thing out of my mouth, and I threw up everywhere. The young nurse asked, and I've *never* forgiven myself for my reply, 'Have you got any problems?' I said, 'For Chrissake, my fucking shoulder is absolutely killing me! I've been trying to tell somebody!' Later we found that in my football career I'd had two very badly damaged shoulders. In opening me up the surgeon had done something to the joint, and that made the pain. I was so *sorry* I went on the way I did at the time. But it was just the way I *felt*. I really had no other feelings of soreness or pain."

In hospital Peter's shoulder became painful too, and it was treated at the time, but, unlike Rick's, his discomfort did not vanish for a year.

"Five days after the operation I had a hell of a pain in my shoulder. When they zip you open, your arm may be anywhere and they're not, I guess, too fussy where. The pain was from my shoulder being virtually dislocated. It's like whiplash and can happen days after they cut you open and pull your ribs to each side. I had no visible bruises. At home I had a physio come. Took a year and it was still painful. I was told by a nurse friend of ours who used to participate in that sort of operation that it wasn't uncommon."

Lachlan had a strange feeling in his foot, and his surgeon showed no interest in it.

"About the fifth day after the operation my left foot was numb, so I reported this to the surgeon, and he said, 'Well, I operated on your *heart*, not your *toe*.' That's all. I had suffered nerve damage, from a chronic bad back, and it may well be that the numb foot wasn't a consequence of the operation but of sitting upright in bed, or it may have been that in turning me on the operating table they banged my back without knowing. Nerve damage became permanent. I have it still."

After the operation Kim's serious difficulties led him to believe that altogether he might have died several times during his 35 days in hospital. He was exhausted and felt poorly immediately after the operation. The nurse acted quickly, and afterwards Kim believed that part of the final operation procedure had to be repeated.

"No energy, couldn't even move my hand. I kept saying there's something wrong. The surgeon came back because people'd said, 'Look, he's in big trouble. We don't think he'll last through the night. Would you tell his wife?' There was a tall male nurse, six foot six inches, I nicknamed him 'Lurch' ... I said, 'I've got a pain here.' And then apparently I *died* again. So Lurch pressed the blue light button, everybody comes, and he gave me CPR. They broke my sternum again, which had only been stitched two days before, and broke all the stainless steel pins."

Breathing problems followed, and after an X-ray the cause was established and Kim's lungs were treated, dramatically.

"They moved me back into the special ward. I was having difficulty breathing all the time. They make you get up and have a shower. I couldn't. The nurse said, 'Yes you can. You're a big strong man. Take your breaths.' So they sent a psychiatrist or a psychologist in, because they believed I should've been able to take the deep breaths. They thought it was *mental*, that I wasn't trying. I tried to explain that I can't breathe. She's saying, 'Yes you can. It's in your mind, just make yourself do it.' The next day she came in and made me go to physiotherapy. She walked me out, and when I went into the room, there were eight patients all doing these exercises. Well, I never went back. Next day the patients asked, 'Did that guy die?' I must've looked like a drowned rat. This went on until the eighth day in hospital. I'm still puffing. My old friend came every day and finally he went the medical registrar and said, 'I know this guy. You're saying to me it's *mental*, that he's not trying to breathe, I know this guy'd be busting his guts to get well.' So they took an X-ray and found in the operation my right lung had collapsed. I'd had that since after the CPR. If you're really fit, you have five litres of air in two lungs. For eight days I had only *two* litres of air. No wonder I couldn't breathe. They came next morning, put a big tube into the top of my ribs and two litres of water goes into a big bowl. I felt terrific, and terrific mentally too! I can now breathe! I can cough!"

Early recovery—ill and drugged

In the ward, recovery from the patient's point of view goes through three stages. The first is dominated by feelings of physical pain, nausea and drug-induced sleep; next you become aware that the illness is passing, the drugs are being withdrawn, pain is turning to discomfort, and there is a scar to prove it all happened. Tubes are removed and you must clear your lungs and begin to walk.

Early recovery can be dominated by feelings associated with pain-killing drugs that make you comfortable—but at a price. Chris endured unexpected bruises.

"On heavy morphine for the first couple of days. I'd go in and out of consciousness, and a few hours later someone would put another needle in. I was in no discomfort. They had a saline drip and a blood plasma drip. But because I am so thin it was so hard for them to find places to put in needles. Often the needle wouldn't stay in, and they had to put it in another spot. My wrists and hands were a mass of bruises from drips and needles. More uncomfortable than the incision."

Lachlan recalled feeling sick as he tried to eat a bowl of soup, and vomiting over a nurse as she rushed up with a towel. Erik, too, felt nauseous, and Kim recalled the embarrassment of being unable to control one's bodily functions.

"Lying in bed, you can't eat, you've just got no energy, and you do some really embarrassing things. You want to go to the toilet but you can't raise the energy, and then all of a sudden the bed's a mess and you can't do anything about it, and then they've got to come and lift you up and clean you, and that was really bad news as far as I was concerned."

Catherine and Hank remembered the hallucinations and nightmares that the drugs gave rise to, although Hank knew that his positive feeling for drugs would not be allowed to last.

"I was realising morphine was pretty good stuff! But they said, 'No more of that. We'll have to give it to you in a suppository this time.' After a couple of *them* I wasn't so keen."

Others felt optimistic about their progress and their ability to carry on without the use of drugs. Brad found that the pain was manageable as he began his recovery.

"I began to recover quicker than I expected. And the pain was good. That sounds funny, doesn't it? It was not excruciating, wasn't really a bad pain."

Chest scar, staples and stitches

Surgeons rejoin the chest at the breastbone, and a livid scar is visible. After a few weeks the scar becomes an accepted part of the body, and its prominence is largely forgotten. Chris recalled the first sight of his scar.

"I had no pyjama jacket on, no covering at all, so I could look down and I could see this red stripe right down me."

Hank wondered why he had no stitches.

"They didn't tell me a lot. I can remember when they pulled the tape off, I was amazed that there were no stitches. Lying in bed on my elbow I felt my sternum go click, click. That's a bad feeling. There were these little wire twitches and they twitch your bones together. They told me that's what they do to your sternum. I always found that a bit of a worry because I wonder where the ends are. I can't feel it."

Lachlan recalled having stitches out, while James still had his staples in.

"The skin's grown over. Your ribs are all joined up at the ends with stainless steel staples. They're still in there, and they can't take them out."

Liam's scar looks like a small scratch. He has faint marks at the bottom of his rib cage where the wire and the drainage tubes were.

"After twelve years the healing is fantastic. It had a happy outcome. My surgeon, she took out a major vein. You'd never know it now. If you look very carefully you can see a bit of scar. They cut about half an inch, and then further along the leg another incision of about half an inch and further along still, another half inch and they just tease the vein out."

However, Barbara found that the scar was placed where it would always concern her.

"I still buy clothes that cover up my scar, and I don't wear much open. It's not a bad scar ... really just a silver line. In fact it improved over the years. I had a little cord down it for a while, but that settled down."

Taking out the tubes

Tubes coming out of your body are taken away before you can move about easily. The respirator tube is usually removed in Intensive Care; the second set of tubes are those that drain the chest and the bladder. While the removal of the respirator tube brings great relief, removal of the second set is accompanied more by surprise than discomfort.

Liam remembered the removal of the tubes as a turning point in his recovery.

"In the transition ward blood pressure monitoring is taken out and they remove the catheter but the drain tubes at the bottom of the chest are still there. And a little bit of metal also comes out. At the conclusion of the operation, they lay a bit of thin wire on the heart and feed it out through the chest wall as they close up the chest, so in the event of the heart needing a restart, they can use the tip of the wire to shock it into activity again. These three things are coming out, the wire and the two drain tubes either side. You're getting in touch with the environment, you're starting to speak to people alongside you, you're saying, 'I'm here I made it!' You're getting a real lift in spirits and talking with the others and saying positive things to one another."

Barbara had the respirator tube taken out after each time she went into surgery, and both times it was most uncomfortable.

"The tube was taken out—that was awful—pulling out the tube I felt I was drowning; and the second time I had the tube come out I felt that awful feeling again."

The task of removing the tubes in the chest is difficult for the nurses to mention or discuss until *after* the event, as Hank discovered.

"You can't do much until they get out the tubes from inside your chest. You've got a catheter for the bladder as well. That was the painful one. When they were going to take the chest tubes out I asked how far they went in. 'Just a couple of inches.' She asks, 'Are you ready?' Then she pulls out about six feet of rubber! Burns like crazy! 'You said it was only an inch!' I said. 'I had to lie to you,' the nurse said, 'or you wouldn't have let me do it! It'll stop hurting in a minute.'"

David, too, was taken by surprise.

"You've got these three things going in under the lower diaphragm. You don't know that they go right up to near your neck at the top of your chest, and when they pull them out you can't believe how much comes out. They don't tell you that—they don't want you to know—because I had the three tubes in and then they went *shshshst!* I thought they'd pull my ears with them! That *was* a big shock. But that took only one second. The nurse thought it was terribly funny."

Physiotherapy and coughing

Once the respirator tube and the draining tubes in your chest are gone you become entirely responsible for your breathing. But this can be difficult because your lungs are partly collapsed, and ugly residue from the operation has to be cleared from them. At this point for Liam, under directions from the surgeon, the physiotherapist became a friend with a cushion.

"On day three the surgeon said tomorrow would be a big day because the drain tubes will be removed, and the muck from your bruised lungs that has been draining out through those tubes won't be able to get out through there, and on day four your lungs will cough it up, and get rid of it. The physio ... said the main thing to do is to hold the pillow tightly even though you feel pain on the chest. 'Don't get worried, because your chest is wired together ... You can't do any damage.' You press quite firmly with the pillow so as to minimise chest wall movement while you're coughing. 'I'm not going to kid you that it's not going to be painful,' she said, 'but you'll be so glad to get rid of the phlegm.' The nurses had come and removed the drain tubes, and soon you start feeling that you want to cough. They turn you on your side, you grab the pillow, they have a basin there, and into it you cough away phlegm out your mouth. You don't swallow it. It's uncomfortable pain. If you try to cheat, and not press hard on the pillow, it does become raw pain."

Lachlan felt the raw pain, felt that his whole body would give way when he had to cough, and believed that no one could prepare for it.

"You feel as though your chest's going to split apart when you cough. I don't know how one can prepare people for the agony of the cough ...

At the time you think your internal organs have given way. I was instructed in how to cough on the day before the operation."

Brad was also puzzled at first by the need to get his chest clear inside, and felt there had not been enough warning or preparation for the exercise to understand its value clearly.

"There is very little depth of information given apart from the physio saying, 'I'll be pushing on you and you'll be wishing I'd go away.' They have a special exercise they wanted you to do mainly, deep breathing, and they show you how to hold onto a little pillow when you cough, and the leg exercise was raising and lowering and bending and just keeping your feet moving."

Walking in hospital

Now you are free of drugs and the nausea that they often produce, and your tubes are gone from the throat and chest. You can breathe properly again, and the physiotherapist now has the task of helping you to begin to walk securely. This is surprising and exhausting at first, but as time passes your body comes back under your control. In learning to walk again, your body is your guide, as Liam found, and when you follow it, confidence is built. Like Liam, Chris learned quickly to take responsibility for walking, while accepting the early support given by his physiotherapist.

"Day three, the physiotherapist came, ran through very simple exercises to keep the chest from collapsing. That afternoon I got up, went to the lavatory, and they said to walk around the corridors as much as you want to. The physiotherapist came with me for the first two times. If I felt a bit unstable I would grab her elbow if the chest pain wasn't too bad. I felt amazingly weak. She said, 'First time we'll go once around the rectangle, then you can go back and have a snooze.' I was very glad to get back and have a snooze. From then on, four walks a day. You really have to regulate yourself according to how you feel."

On the other hand, James found walking was not what he wanted to do.

"Oh boy, you don't really want to walk. You don't think you can possibly do it. Two people hold you and you really feel your whole body's going to fall apart."

Others found walking easy, but it was a personal battle at first for Catherine. Then she discovered she was recovering rapidly, and that unanticipated difficulties on the way were her responsibility.

"I was amazed at the recovery. First I could have half an hour in a chair, as if it were a reward for something! I was terrified I was going to fall and hurt myself. I begged to be put back into bed. Utterly at the mercy of others. But then I realised that today was so much better than yesterday. After being this lady at the mercy of the world, full of agony and fear, I was shuffling to the bathroom, hanging onto beds. On the fourth day I got out of the ward, across the corridor, to a big triangular pillar called 'the mulberry bush'. The idea was to go around the mulberry bush and come back. I got to the pillar and collapsed. They pushed a wheelchair underneath me and got me back into bed. Poor physiotherapist was doing this for me, and I threw up all over her! She explained to me that was not *my* problem. It was *hers*, she should have ducked. She explained to me that when the heart beats madly like it does against the stomach, it has repercussions on the stomach muscles. The next day I made it around the mulberry bush and came back. I was in for eight days, and each time I was walking further."

Rick, too, knew he needed help to walk at first, was surprised at how rapidly he recovered. On the other hand, Peter worked independently, made walking a challenge, and hurried to leave hospital as soon as possible.

"I used to go out on the terrace about half past six in the morning and then come back, and sometimes complain about the hospital's lack of maintenance. I used to walk round and round and round and round because I wanted to get out of the place. I knew I had to show I could walk so I just put my dressing gown on and walked. Came out eight days later. They got tired of me walking round and round the ward, trying to prove I was fit."

8

In the ward—later recovery

The final stage in your hospital recovery, the stage when you really feel you are regaining control of life, centres on eating and using the toilet, washing yourself and thinking about getting home, entertaining yourself and taking an interest in others. When you entered hospital you might have had a choice of a private room or a public ward for your recovery.

Private rooms and visitors

Would it be better to have a room to yourself, or go into a ward with other people? When you complete the hospital's application form, you are asked whether or not you want a private room, and you are told that if you do, it is not always possible to provide one at the time you expect it. So unless you have special public duties and privileges, like those of a senior politician, or can otherwise influence the hospital's administration, you may not be able to determine the accommodation you have during recovery. In many communities, taking out private health insurance is in itself not enough to get a private room. Peter had a private room because, first, one was available, and second, as a matter of course, his name was high on the list because he had been a generous foundation member of the hospital.

Some people imagine that they would be better suited to a public ward because they like the company of other people, but Chris didn't want the company of other patients or their conversation.

"Didn't meet other patients in the same situation. It was never suggested that I went to a post-operative group to talk about my recovery. If it had been suggested, I would've declined. I'm too private a person for that sort of thing."

Erik did not want to share a room either, because he found other people's visitors were tiresome.

"You're in pain, and on the third day I got my private room, which I liked because you feel total and utter exhaustion. All you want is sleep ... Trouble is when visitors come. Four people each. Sixteen people in that little room! When you don't feel well, that is punishment. 'Sh, sh, sh' all the time. You can go crazy. When I got my own room that really helped."

On the other hand, James could not have imagined himself in anything but a shared ward. He wanted to hear of the experiences of other patients, to feel secure in their company and learn about differing recovery rates from them.

"I would never go into hospital and have a room by myself, because if anything's wrong someone can alert other people. In a room by yourself I'd be absolutely terrified that you wouldn't know what was happening, or when it was happening. You find out things that you don't even know what to ask about ... And you actually *see* people *recovering*. You learn so much as you see people recovering. You progress, and can see other people progressing."

Liam felt ambivalent about having a private room. At first he did not want to be disturbed by the unknown habits of patients or interruptions from hospital staff. But at the end of his hospital stay, being a person who liked the company of others, he realised that this was not as good an idea as he had imagined.

"In retrospect, it probably would've been better if I *hadn't* had a private room. I liked being in a private room because I could just order my own existence. It's got your own en suite and you can sleep without being inter-rupted except the nurse coming in. You don't have to make conversation with people or their visitors. When you're not feeling up to it you really don't want to."

Food and entertainment

In the last stage of recovery you regain control of your own welfare. You want to eat, taste food, and use the bathroom. Chris had a standing order for two dozen oysters and was happy to know he had to drink as much as possible. After six days Peter found the food he was given had no flavour, and wanted something with taste, so his wife went for a pizza. She got it, but he found it was not what interested him. He even thought he wanted a Scotch whisky. His wife brought him a whole bottle, but he didn't want that either.

"I enjoy food. If the food doesn't taste I'm not interested. The first meal I had in hospital I said, 'What the hell have you done to this? It's dreadful.' They said, 'Oh well, there's no salt because most people are on a no-salt diet.' I said, 'Well, I'm not.' In fact I'd lost my taste. But it was all right by the end of the week."

It took Erik two days before any interest in food returned. Lachlan could not remember exactly when he began to eat food again, but Liam was eating by day four.

"On day four I was starting to eat properly. On day three, pretty light sort of stuff, and day four starting to get food, and the dietitian came in and discussed the next day's menu with me."

In time it becomes necessary to be entertained in hospital. With this operation there are limits to the kind of entertainment you can have. Peter enjoyed a comfortable chair, TV and a book, all the entertainment he wanted. Unlike Peter, Chris found that he couldn't get the entertainment he had expected in reading. Erik liked TV amusements, and suffered from his sense of humour.

"They've got the TV above you. I watched a funny movie and I started laughing and I turned it off quickly, it hurt like hell … one thing you can't do is laugh."

Showering

Being able to take a shower alone was a great forward step, and Chris remembered it for the help nurses offered. Barbara also remembered her helpful nurses, largely because of their high expectations.

> "Forty-eight hours after the operation they said, 'Right! Time to have shower!' They gave me a plastic chair in the shower. I ran the shower, bathed myself. No stiffness in the shoulders. I didn't suffer from the strain of opening your rib cage. The muscles in my back were sore because of cutting of the nerves. Next day I asked for a chair. 'No, you don't get a chair this time.' I had to shower standing up! They get you moving very quickly."

When Catherine had her shower she took her drips in with her.

> "About day three I used the shower, and went to the lavatory, but you had to take everything with you, drips on wheels, and all that came along with it. The nurse showered me. I couldn't possibly have showered alone. I sat on the seat and she showered and dried me. Somehow I summoned enough energy to get back to bed and slept for an hour or so. Very enervating."

Going home?

The time you spend recovering in hospital is determined by the particular doctor who is in charge of your operation. They decide when you are well enough to go home. There are rules, but problems can arise. After seven days in hospital, Lachlan learned the rules of how to judge when a patient was ready to go home.

> "They have a rule that they won't let you out until you can go along the corridor, down one flight of steps, along a corridor, up two flights of steps onto the roof of the building, walk round the roof, and walk back to your bed, unaided. Do that and you're fit to go home, under the supervision of a loved one."

Hank, relatively young for this operation, was put in a room with older men, where the rule was not related to climbing stairs but on a first-in-first-out basis. But in Hank's case it appeared that the medical staff had a different rule, and, because he seemed so young and fit, they presented him with a personal problem.

> "The medical staff thought, 'This guy's a young fit one. We'll see if we can get him out in two days.' I was cooperating with them for a bit, and then I thought, 'Hang on a second, I'm not going to go out like *this*.' I kicked up a

bit. I did not want to go. They did me on the Monday and they wanted to get me out by the Thursday. Four days! Ridiculous. I said, 'Hey, I'm not *ready* to go.' There wasn't anyone at home. They said they'd keep me until Monday. But by the time Saturday came, I rang my parents and they came and picked me up and I went home."

Kim, like Hank, was almost sent home too soon as well.

"Doctor said, 'You can go home tomorrow.' Well, that really put me down because I knew that I couldn't've gone anywhere tomorrow. I couldn't breathe. There was no way I could go. I didn't want to stay in hospital, but I couldn't go anywhere else. When my friend came that night I said, 'I can't go home.' He said, 'You're not going home.' I said that the doctor told me I was going home. And he hauled that young doctor over the coals because he hadn't read the card properly."

However, Rick was overjoyed to be going home after a very short stay of seven days.

"My surgeon said, 'You can thank your mental attitude and your physical fitness level for getting you through so quickly … Tell your wife to come and get you in the morning.' That was special, really special."

Barbara had eight days in hospital and came home to a comforting welcome.

"I stayed at home the first day and a half. Some neighbour brought round a meal. Then my husband had to go away for the weekend. So I went to the golf club and stayed there. Didn't need any nursing care. Didn't have to get up for breakfast. Showered and dressed when I was ready, lunch was laid on at the restaurant. I walked in the garden, gentle walks on the flat. And a friend came the first day … Next day a couple more friends came, and when my husband came back he stayed at the club for another day or two. That had set me up. It was wonderful."

$$\bigodot{9}$$

Rehabilitation

After your heart surgery, the medical staff attach great value to your diet and exercise. The hospital gives you medical literature, dieticians have advice for you, and physiotherapists have exercises that are vital to recovery. Much technical advice is available from the National Heart Foundation, which provides the most recent technical information on recovery and rehabilitation after heart surgery. There are also extension programs run by hospitals and community rehabilitation centres. You have a choice. Recover and rehabilitate yourself alone, or in the company of others.

Some people find the company of others a great help; they can judge their own recovery by comparison with others, and they can get helpful tips. On the other hand, because the recovery–rehabilitation process is unique and personal, it can become an intensely private matter, and competing or comparing oneself with others might not be acceptable. By this stage you feel the operation has been a success, and your recovery is under way, and you recover in unpredictable bursts in uncertain ways, and achieve different goals.

Exercise classes

Informants had differed in their views of diets and exercises. David followed the medical advice precisely, while Hank and Kim ignored it.

In the hospital David went to exercise classes and, after going home, would walk half a kilometre from home to the hospital to more classes run by the hospital's outside program.

"They touched on food, exercise, non-smoking, getting yourself dressed, and making home ready for you ... Twenty people were in each session, one a week for six weeks. There was one man in his forties, me in my fifties, and everyone else was in their sixties to eighties ... When I got there they said that everyone had to walk around the passageways. I'd already walked from home. But some people couldn't even walk the passageways. I was able to wheel the supermarket trolley, carry all the weights, and go up and down the steps, and do all that was necessary. I went to four of the sessions."

Hank felt that the rehabilitation classes in the hospital were not informative, and believed that he was fit enough not to need any help from rehabilitation classes outside hospital.

"They want you to go to counselling, but I didn't do that. They wanted me to do exercise classes, but I didn't want to do them. They gave me a folder of stuff. Wasn't necessary because I lead an active lifestyle anyway. I wasn't going to go classes with a lot of 70-year-old ladies! Nutrition classes weren't telling me anything I didn't already know."

On the other hand, Liam learned much from the exercise program conducted at the hospital and thought it suitable for people at home.

"A cardiac rehabilitation nurse told me about a rehabilitation program. Met on Wednesday morning at the hospital for six weeks for education in diet, exercise and relaxation. I went. Appropriate information was put in a way the lay person had no trouble with it. They checked to see the audience were getting the message. Relevant, very interactive, and they encouraged people to ask questions and voice their concerns ... They had exercises for arms, legs, and the body, all appropriate for post-op recovery. They told you what you could do at home, and how often. I was impressed."

Brad had had two heart operations and felt that although the classes might be necessary they were not anything to look forward to.

"I went to post-operative classes after the first operation at the hospital once a week for at least a month. Walking around, up steps, down steps, various exercises, discussion, meditation, relaxation. Not the second time I had an operation. It *was* good for you, but I wasn't sorry to stop. I got a little bit tired of people dwelling on their own illness, and I got bored doing exactly the same thing. Not very joyful. But it served a function. Gave you a bit of a pick-me-up, a mental stimulus, a bit of a kick along."

Barbara was half-hearted towards classes, and although Kim went to rehabilitation he too found, largely because he was no longer willing to be in hospital, that organised classes had little to offer him.

James thought that the collapse of his lung during the operation had made him feel very tired. Medical staff suggested he do breathing exercises, and attend hospital rehabilitation classes after he was discharged.

"I did go to exercise classes and I did take up swimming because they said that's good exercise. I went to those classes at the YMCA and for about eighteen months, twice a week. That sort of trailed off because I'm not naturally a swimmer."

Diet

Erik had no need of expert advice on diet because he and his wife simply adhered to their well-established low-cholesterol diet. On the other hand, both Liam and David learned much from attending rehabilitation sessions about diet.

"The rehabilitation exercise classes were good and so was a talk by one expert I knew personally on what you eat and don't eat. They had tapes of him. The one thing that stuck in my mind was, 'Don't eat eggs. What you should do is—if you are going to eat eggs—take the yolk out and give it to your dog. Let *him* have the heart attack, and *you* eat the whites.'"

Peter learned about proper diet from an acquaintance with heart disease and followed the advice closely, with occasional lapses. He also went to group meetings in hospital, and practised carefully what he had learned.

"In hospital the cardiac patients met in a small group to talk about what one should eat. They also had a group on psychological aspects ... The only thing I ever heard is that you might suffer depression ... I learned what I should and shouldn't eat, basically to do with cholesterol. When I first knew something was wrong I think my cholesterol was about 8. I got down to 6.6. I'd like it down below 6. But I don't think my cardiologist is too worried. My blood pressure's something like 130/80. It seems to me that's probably your best indicator. You shouldn't eat a lot of animal fat, but if you go out to dinner, *splurge*, it doesn't matter ... we don't eat as much meat as we used to. I don't eat anywhere near as much cheese ... We eat fish, quite a lot of pasta. Virtually given up bacon and eggs. Love it but I know I shouldn't and we cut down our egg intake. Of course, they've changed their mind about that now ... Honestly, I don't do anything as far as my heart is concerned, except have a reasonable diet and try to exercise, keep fit, and get rid of some of the weight. Hopefully you feel a bit more comfortable. Won't make you live any longer."

Like Peter, Kim would also splurge occasionally, always comforting himself with the knowledge that he was no heavier now than in his sporting days, and still is the character he always liked to be.

"I'm 60 and I weigh the same as I weighed when I played football. And I eat good food, but I splurge and have chocolate eclairs. But you are what you are."

Exercising at home

Erik and David took exercise charts home. They felt the instructions must be followed religiously, and saw great improvements in their well-being. Hank was told not to use his car for three weeks; but he drove it down to the local fishing jetty, where he started playing around with his boat. Chris was very pleased to get home, largely because he loathed hospital life. While Kim and Barbara found coming home was all they could have wished for, each managed their recovery quite differently. She took gentle walks, while he felt driven to high activity.

"Two weeks later I was back to work. I bought an exercise bike and had a treadmill delivered. I've still got a farm up the country but I don't use it as much as I used to, but I will now. I take the dog for a walk down the beach on flat ground, and I walk as fast as my mates. If I walk up a hill I can feel the heart rate coming, so I don't exert myself. I swim at the local pool with three of my mates one night a week. They swim a kilometre while I'd swim 400 metres. I just pace it along, stop at the end, there's no race. I enjoy it instead ... although I did swim in the winter swimming club championships in '98 ... 25 metres in a very fast time, but I couldn't walk or talk afterwards. That was stupidity. I was being an egotist, because I was with a lot of my mates, and I didn't want to look an idiot. I was a good swimmer when I was younger. And they didn't know I'd had a heart attack."

Barbara went to the other extreme.

"I was given a list of when I could do this, that, and the other. Couldn't drive for five weeks ... I could get up and down steps as soon as I walked out of the hospital. That surprised me. I thought there'd be a limit on that, and there wasn't. I was told I could play tennis at eight weeks. I couldn't chop wood until twelve weeks after the operation. I played tennis in the eleventh week, and felt like a kid with a new toy!"

Both James and Lachlan found the early days at home were not enjoyable or easy. James found that it took him ages to be able to walk. Rick went to exercise classes, where he was amazed at how tired he felt.

"At exercise class they gave you a chart with additional exercises as you got better. I was exhausted the first time I went ... When you got home there were exercises to be done twice a day, sit-ups and stretches, standing up and sitting down, standing with a chair. These were strenuous. You had to do a certain number in a certain time. I would finish them, but I'd be so *tired* afterwards."

Lachlan was busy recovering as soon as he arrived home, but like the others found that he collapsed by the end of the day, and was shattered by a chest cold. Catherine recovered well, but not before being terrified by the question, How do I manage my life?

"First I went to stay with my youngest daughter, then I had two weeks with my eldest daughter. Otherwise I would have gone to a rehabilitation centre. The first night was terrifying. There was no one. I couldn't ring a bell in the night if I needed any information. My daughter was wonderful, but she wouldn't have the knowledge. I began to notice things that I didn't notice in hospital. Strange feelings in the chest. But in the light of day it didn't seem as terrifying. Next day I went to the local doctor and he was very re-assuring. I was on pain-killers for three weeks for discomfort in the wound. Then I woke up one day, and I didn't need any pain-killer in the morning, didn't need any in the afternoon, and I'd gone all day without them. I had some that night. Suddenly I didn't need them any more!"

(10)

Life after a bypass

How long should you be away from work? Two weeks? Three months? Medical advice appears to favour about two to three months; but how much time you need to rest will be given by the specialist. Their decision is the best you can get. Whether or not you follow it is for you to decide. Among the informants, that decision varied according to their lifestyle, personality, experience of pain, the need for drugs, domestic activities, and the feeling that activity at work is better than restlessness at home

What do you do after having a heart bypass and you feel you are recovering? Some people make changes around the home so that they can manage to move items and do their housework easily. You will begin to see yourself through the eyes of the family, friends and acquaintances who feel you need their help. Perhaps you will change your habits: recognise and accept the ageing of your body and that you cannot alter that process, except by ceasing to smoke and to eat fatty foods; manage your physical welfare with regular, light exercise by giving up running for walking, tennis for golf, and arguments for listening. Again, the decision is yours: reduce life's excitements, increase them, or take up easier distractions that you like?

What you choose to do depends largely on how you see yourself. Some informants saw great changes in themselves, others refused to do so. Some felt their memory falter, their creativity wane, and vagueness extend itself. Old age, or the shock of the operation? Big things appeared to be heavier, and the need for physical help became clear. Speech could change. Some people felt a great blow to their confidence, embarrassed by being less a person because of heart disease, while others were vulnerable to threats that earlier they would have scorned. Anger rose among the relatives who were not warned that a heart patient may briefly have a change of character. Again, you decide for the sake of yourself how the shock of surgery will take you. You will not always be conscious of its effects. You may, if you choose, refuse to be depressed, and manage your affairs as if nothing much had happened to you; or you might take a little more time to shift responsibilities onto others, and manage your affairs differently.

Back to work

Some informants returning to work or home activities felt alienated, that they were not what they had been, or that they wanted to change the way they had been. Going back to work was important to several men—more so than the women—and appeared to relate to plans to either retire, meet some prearranged scheme or capture work's therapeutic effects.

Lachlan had arranged to be back at his university at an agreed time after the operation. There were no medical complications to prevent the arrangement; it was simply a matter of returning from sick leave.

"I was back at work within nine weeks of the operation. Other people I know got back much quicker, but I had made an arrangement to return at a certain time if all was well."

Unlike Lachlan, James was away from work a little longer than expected. He became concerned about his diet and prescribed drugs, saw his doctor regularly, and slowly got back to his normal activities.

"I had three months off before I went back to work. Wife was just looking after me at home, very supportive, terrific, and really concerned about putting me on a very strict diet with small quantities. When you go home they give you a whole lot of drugs. For pain over about ten days, and to make the blood thin I took aspirin ... At least three months before I could drive. Moving your chest makes it an effort to park."

Brad went back to work after two months; Chris, who had retired several years before the operation, worked preparing his sailboat; Peter returned to work with his wife in their travel business in their own offices at home, while Brad and Kim went back to work as soon as they felt like it, probably too soon in Kim's case.

"Take two months off? Never! That's probably my personality problem. I don't sit, I'm an active person. If my brain was telling me I was feeling good, and I had the energy to walk, why would I want to sit at home? Went against medical advice, but I was bored at home, and I just figured I could do more at work."

Rick, too, found that all he wanted was to get back to his business. He was alone at home, he had no one to talk to, no interest in gardening, and, like Kim, was not one to sit down and read books. Determined to get back into shape fast, he decided to do many more exercises than required. Still feeling frustrated and agitated, he behaved as if he were not recovering at home but back at work full-time.

"We live in a rural area on an acre, so there are no next-door neighbours. I was agitated and sad because I was pinned down. I am the founder of the business, major shareholder, and I was concerned you can't have much time away. I got a fax machine, worked via the office. Making phone calls, doing deals. I had ideas. The business went on. That helped me. Couldn't drive. Think of that! Been in sales and marketing all my life. People were busy and couldn't come and see me. I couldn't have any visitors. I used to break my neck for the Monday and the Thursday exercise classes, to see the other guys. We all had our operations at the same time. And then I'd get a cab home. They told me after the operation that I could expect to be away for three months. But I felt well enough not to be. That's what frustrated me. I did probably twice the number of exercises—because it gave me something to do. Not a gardener, tried reading books. And I even cooked!"

A new lifestyle

Maintaining a new level of health led the informants to reassess what activities were appropriate to their new life. Some took life quietly, others became reflective about their style of living, and a few decided that taking firm control of life and a high level of activity were best.

Catherine feels better since her operation, rests when she feels like it, has returned to teaching and, with help from her daughters and someone to do heavy housework, she can maintain her home without great effort.

"I don't have any tiredness, and feelings of weakness that I had before. I had to get someone in to do the vacuuming ... I have small steps to reach things up high. I don't keep heavy things high up. In the shower there's a bar in the wall, and a non-slip mat in the bath. If it's cold, and I've got the fire on, I nod off for an hour or so in the afternoon. I look after myself. My children have been so caring ... When I got back into circulation at University of the Third Age—I tutor in gardening and history—I would move my chair and someone would rush over saying, 'Don't do this. Don't do that!' Luckily my family are not like that. They know I have enough sense, that I wouldn't do something if I couldn't."

Rick looks after his health carefully and, finding that he has no health problems, takes a new approach to his activities.

"I have regular checks, I walk and sleep well, and I have learned a lesson. I don't get wound up and as stressed as much as I used to. Life is to be lived. Whereas things used to annoy me, now I take action."

At his new level of health, Peter's major activity is walking, and he seems to have no ill effects from the operation.

"Took it easy for a few weeks. Lifting, carrying, moving, was no different than it was before the operation because of my back injury. Now it's mainly stretching. My wife and I walk every morning before breakfast for anything from three to six kilometres, for my back, nothing to do with my heart. Quite honestly I don't do *anything* as far as my heart is concerned. Except a reasonable diet and exercise to keep fit. It gets rid of some of the weight, just keeps you generally fit, and hopefully you feel a bit more comfortable as long as you live. It won't make you live any longer. Other people some-times have a pain in their chest. Mine was just numb. I really had no feeling in it for six months."

Shortly after the operation Chris hoped that he, too, would feel better and was looking forward to an active life. But he grew tired and weak, and had to curtail his activities. The pain in his chest severely limited exercising. Breathing was restricted and, although nothing seemed the matter with his limbs, he walked with difficulty, and could not lift and carry items easily.

> "The post-hospital pain in my whole upper structure was much greater than in hospital. I couldn't keep straight except when I did my exercises. I had to go back to a hunched position. The first walks were so dreadful, every step jerked my wound. At first I had to walk like a little old man with tiny steps, hunched over, otherwise when I breathed in, severe pain went right throughout the rib cage. It was three months before I could drive the car. Much longer than I'd anticipated. I couldn't even travel *in* a car before more than two weeks, because I couldn't manage the physical movement. Nothing wrong with the wrists, elbows or hands. Just couldn't lift anything. I suppose I got stronger."

Ethan found recently that only one of the three blood vessels treated originally was fully open. His specialist would not recommend having the operation again, and Ethan agrees that at the age of 82 it is hardly worthwhile. He enjoys golf, uses a golf buggy, and takes prescribed medication to prevent blood clotting.

> "I play golf on a handicap of 21. I use a golf cart because I could not walk around the golf course. I walk all right on the flat, but going uphill, I have troubles. I get angina and use Nitrolingual ... At my age you can't expect to do the things you were doing at 70, much less the things you were doing at 50."

Hank has reduced the exertion he puts into recreation, is aware of ageing and of being occasionally out of breath, and has changed his attitude to the major sources of tension in life.

> "I don't swim. I'm not surfing as much as I used to. I play tennis once a week. I don't have any problems, except I still get short of breath. But that comes with getting older, and going a bit too hard. I just don't worry. I don't argue. If my kids are wanting to do stuff that I don't agree with, and they are getting out of hand, I just let them do it. They survive."

Over the last three years at home, David curtailed his regular activities and changed habits that he felt were not going to help him stay well. He does not smoke, and believes he eats more fatty foods than he should, but comforts himself with the idea that others tell him he can eat fatty food 'just this once'. He has no ailments, he is not overweight, he swims, he works half a day and walks for the rest of the day, and does not feel anything except the line of the 'zip' down the centre of his chest. By comparison with a friend who had the operation twelve years ago, David thinks he is better off, but does worry about how long he's got to live. Tennis has been dropped and golf is his game.

> "When you play golf you've got two hands together on the club, so you feel you are protecting your chest. The difference with tennis is you are not protecting your chest. You are hitting with your central chest muscles ... Psychologically I think, 'Oh, I don't want to do that.' I know I *can*. But I haven't *done* it. I just think my days of tennis are over."

James takes life quietly, but for some time he was concerned about how long the operation would affect his activities.

> "I still get tired but I think it's old age now. If I say I'm tired, someone always points out that I've been doing such and such and comments, 'You can expect to be tired.' What terrifies me is that no one knows how long it would last ... If I got five years out of it, that'd be good. It's been ten. I've been on a very low fat diet and I play golf and walk every day for half an hour. I must admit I've walked less since I've been working at my new library. I do a fair bit of gardening."

There was nothing that Kim, a self-confessed hedonist, would not do. He catalogued a full life and lived it.

> "I feel sensational. I run, I swim, I ride horses, I do all the things that normal people do. My brain is agile, and being a hedonist, I've had an amazing life ... If I died tomorrow I would have no regrets in life. I don't have any problems, and I've been dead twice. I've always believed that if you think healthy, and you keep your brain going, when your number comes up ... that's the story. My use-by date is getting closer. I took up smoking again after about six months. I figured, look, I've had a great life. I'll go, but I'll go the way I want to go. I don't want to be where everybody's doing things for me ... I cook beautiful meals, I get my mates to come round ... I eat good food, but I still would have, on odd occasions, Kentucky Fried Chicken, a glass of red wine with it. I sit and relax ... but at the end of the day I could get hit by a truck."

Changes in feelings about oneself

The operation may affect not only how you feel about your body but also your sense of self. The feelings range from noticeable effects on mental skills and abilities, feelings of sadness and some-times depression, a sense of vulnerability, and an old feeling of dependence.

Brad felt that because he had had so many operations his brain was greatly affected by the anaesthetic, and he did not know whether or not this experience was related to heart disease. He did not feel that he was becoming depressed, but found that his ability to think clearly and effectively had been marred.

> "My brain is nowhere near as effective as it was before, given the number of anaesthetics I've had. Whether it's related to the heart I don't know, but I'm certainly not nearly as quick as I was. I'm forgetting things … They warned me about going too hard."

Although he believed his body recovered well from the opera-tion, Hank thought it had knocked him about psychologically, affecting his view of himself, at work and at home. Also when working alone on his boat he thought carefully about his physical capabilities.

> "I recovered pretty well. Psychologically it knocks you about. I remember being embarrassed about going back to work because of what had happened to me. I remember thinking, 'This is a heart attack. Imagine how someone who has had a psychological breakdown must feel, coming back to face people.' It was strange because these were the people who cared for me, my friends. My wife would say my memory's not as good as it was, that I'm more irritable … You do really lose your confidence. I can understand some people getting depressed. I feel a bit vaguer. I do have trouble grasping things but I think I've always had trouble like that … Might be because I'm getting older. That's my excuse. I'm still being careful about things. I had to pull a big heavy battery out of my boat this morning. Before the heart attack I would've done it on my own. But today I got someone to help me."

Barbara seemed to be free of depression, in spite of a long-standing concern that she wouldn't live long. But she did find her creativity and concentration were marred for a long time.

"Nobody mentioned that they thought I was not myself, but that idea gave me a little insight about my creative patchwork. That interest faded. I still attended club meetings, but I couldn't concentrate for about eighteen months or two years. I didn't have that urge to do patchwork for about two years. At my six weeks review with the surgeon ... I wrote, 'I feel as if I've been given life over again.' To me all the questions looked on the down side. Your body isn't perfect. I once had to face up to being a diabetic so the heart problem didn't have the same effect."

Peter's wife commented on how her husband's body seemed to have changed. She did not understand the changes at the time, but thought they might relate to his breathing and his voice. She also said that Peter could not stay in bed because he had difficulty lying down. This was evident when he was in hospital, and it may have appeared to the medical staff to be related to his apparent impatience. But to her this was not so.

"At the time, it wasn't that noticeable, but since then I have noticed his voice has gone down to a much lower range. When he speaks I often don't hear what he says. Sometimes up, sometimes down. If he's animated, or wants me to hear, then I do hear. But if he's just sitting in the chair, and turns round and says something to me, and I'm across the room, I'm really not sure what he says. It seems his voice went down a bit, and he couldn't get enough oxygen. He still complains about that. He can't lie in a bed. He's not impatient, but rather he has very little time for people who linger around and malinger."

Chris had anticipated some depression after the operation and thought it normal. Many serious complications followed his bypass operation, which gave good reason for feeling in low spirits.

"I was pretty depressed at times. The book that the hospital gave me said it's common. I had just escaped dying, and suddenly realised that you are held together by the miracles of modern surgery. I didn't like seeing many people and couldn't be bothered talking. I am sure that's normal. I would have thought on a scale from zero to ten I would have been somewhere about five."

The operation affected Erik more deeply than the prostate operation he had had years before. He had felt vulnerable, and this depressed him. The feeling passed, and he hoped that he would live another five years.

"I felt a bit down according to my wife ... Probably it's the first time in your life that you feel you are extremely vulnerable. I guess that's probably why people become depressed. It must've been a passing feeling because we never had a problem with it. I slept a lot. But the doctor told me, 'You might feel down a bit. Don't take any tablets or any uppers, just ignore it and you'll feel all right again.' And he was right. If I can have eighty-two years that'll do."

Although he was not fully aware of it, Ethan became depressed, and was a changed person. He did not make a fuss about it himself, and it did not last for very long. His wife felt that there should have been some warning of deep personal changes. Ethan himself appeared to know about the changes, and recalled that they had been unexpected.

"The pamphlet I was given didn't say anything about a change of personality. The patient concerned doesn't know anything about it. I don't think there *was* a great upheaval. Perhaps there was as far as my wife was concerned, and perhaps I was a bit difficult for a while. We went away on a trip and then we were different people. Difficulties passed away pretty soon. If you landed at home on your *own* it would be serious."

Ethan's wife did not meet the heart specialist, and thought she should have been warned about how the operation might affect her husband personally.

"The surgeon never told me anything beforehand. But when I rang he then said, 'Oh, you should have known.' I said, 'How *was* I to know?' And he said, 'When a heart is taken out, and dealt with and put back, that is a most traumatic experience for a body, and will take a little bit longer to adjust.' He didn't tell me how long, but that I had to be more patient. I thought I *was* patient. I felt I wasn't living with the man I knew before he went to hospital. My husband was worried about his eyesight. On the pamphlet it said not to worry if your eyesight's poor. 'Don't go to your oculist. That will eventually right itself.' It did after we began the trip to Bali."

Kim would never allow himself to be depressed. A colourful, active, ebullient character, he found most of the people he knew who had had a heart bypass operation did undergo some changes in the way they felt about themselves. Kim fought feelings of depression. He went to talk to a friend who suffered from depression and declared him a victim of morbidity, looking for excuses to be miserable.

Liam also had a positive approach to the operation and felt he was now in much better health. This was achieved psychologically, and through proper diet and exercise.

"It was good to be rescued from death or a serious restriction, and restored to a life of full activity, without the Sword of Damocles hanging over my head. Just fantastic! You feel so much better. You are able to be active. Some of that is no doubt because of the diet. For years you've been going downhill because of this mucky diet, clogging up arteries. Of course, you are on a high from the endorphins released from your exercise anyway."

Like Hank, David had a business to return to. He had run a hotel without ever worrying how he would deal with drinkers misbehaving at the hotel bar, but now he feels he must be careful. He does not feel depressed, but is learning something new about himself.

"I've run my hotel for as long as I can remember, and I've had no fear of drunks, hoons, anyone at all. But since I've had my operation I feel vulnerable. I have this warning light go on if there's a fight in the bar and someone should be thrown out. I say to myself, 'Hang on a minute. You shouldn't be doing this.' If the hotel staff have any problems now, they tell me to go away. I'm concerned about whether I can actually grab someone, hold them, and put them out. I've never felt vulnerable in my life. It's to do with age, but it was triggered by the operation. My wife says, 'You're crazy. You got to realise you can't do what you did when you were younger.' I don't think stress is going to do me any good. So I dismiss things. I am much easier at work than I was. If there's a problem, I say, 'There's a problem.' Before, if there was a problem, I'd get uptight, until I got it solved. I'm happier to delegate some of my work or authority to somebody in authority. Ten years ago that would never happen. In the traffic also I feel vulnerable."

Catherine, too, found her confidence weaken by having to be so dependent on others.

"You have to rely on other people *so much*. I have been alone so long that I do many things for myself. To have to rely on other people is a dreadful blow to my confidence. I couldn't drive the car. Within two weeks at home I was itching to get into the car. I couldn't even try the steering wheel. It was about six weeks before I could drive again."

Like David and Kim, Rick felt dependent for his life on the close tie he had with his business, and found that not being able to work for so many weeks raised a deep personal problem. He loathed being dependent on others and responded by making a nuisance of himself. However unhappy he felt, Rick learned that the time he spent away from work established in him a new work style both he and his employees preferred.

"My wife will tell you I was not myself, an absolute nuisance in her mind. Very demanding and agitated. Why? I was not allowed to drive for three months ... I was grounded, and she was working—I wanted her to work anyway—but I didn't want her to be *running around* for me. I was being very difficult to live with, and I didn't know it, because that's not me, and she knew it wasn't me. It was happening in the recovery processes, and I didn't understand it. I was making her *really unhappy*. She was caring for me, and I was snapping at the kids. I was at the house and there was nobody there. I was annoying people at the office by calling in to say, 'Why don't we do this, how was that going?' They wanted to be left alone to prove they could run the business, and could show I wasn't necessary. I am not sure that made me feel good. I guess my personality must have done something. Good thing was it gave me a different outlook. I don't get agitated about silly things any more. Somebody's ten minutes late. What am I getting upset about? They are late because they've got a problem. Now at work I feel that I am closer to my employees."

$$\textbf{(11)}$$

Challenges, recovery rate, and advice

Tests, challenges, and projects

Some informants believed that they hastened their recovery by setting themselves tests or challenges and planning projects to advance
their well-being. These included schemes about how they would
manage when they returned home, the study of changes to their
body, and even adventures that would test their recovery.

Erik was impatient with his recovery because he felt tired and
could do nothing about it. A disciplined person, he did his exercises
at home, walked around the tennis court every day, and then tested
himself by taking his wife on a holiday.

> "The first time I walked three to four laps of the tennis court. Then it
> became eight laps, ten laps and you could feel the difference. The operation
> was at the end of March 1994, and by early July we were on our way to a
> holiday in the tropics. Fine, no problems, lovely."

David arranged many projects for himself; refurbishing his large
hotel by dividing it into apartments, building a seaside home, and
taking a trip to Tuscany. His next challenge was to walk up Uluru
(Ayers Rock) in Central Australia. He had done it two years before
the operation and found it difficult. Would it be easier for him to do
it now?

> "I decided I am going to do Ayers Rock. Why? We went about two years
> before the operation. At one stage I was lying on my back, exhausted. My

wife was nowhere near as exhausted as I was, and she was saying I was weak, a slacker. We got to the top. The hardest thing I'd done in my life. That was a test, and it affected me then. I'd like to see now if it was as hard as I remember. My wife often says, 'You're lucky. You could've had a heart attack doing that.'"

Rick was very fit after the rehabilitation exercises, but he still wanted to get back to his business. It survived well without him for three months. What should he do? He needed action. The operation had been done in April, it was winter now, so he decided to take a holiday to test his fitness. Where? Like David, he believed he was well enough to climb Uluru.

"At the end of the rehabilitation period you'd be an Olympian, if you did it properly. I received my certificate, top of the class, felt pretty chuffed. But sitting at home was a waste of time. I wanted to go somewhere warm … I said to my wife, 'Darling, wouldn't it be an accomplishment to have had open-heart surgery, and to climb Ayers Rock. Because people *die* on Ayers Rock. And I feel so *great* now. Wouldn't it be something *special* to do?' She agreed. At Ayers Rock it's sunrise, the Rock is changing colours, and … I said to my daughter, 'Come on. We're going to climb it.' 'No you're not, Dad!' I started to walk towards the Rock. My wife got out of the car screaming. I hadn't done it to upset her. It was just that I was going to do it. My daughter said she'd come. We got to the point where there's a chain to hold on to, and we didn't go any further. We stood at the chain, and said, 'Enough is enough. I've been on Ayers Rock.' I stopped at that point, saying to myself, 'This is stupid, crazy.' So we just sat there and took some photographs. Then we went to Broome, swam in the surf and the warm water. That was where I really I came to peace."

Liam walks 30 minutes daily and rides an exercise bike watching television. But, like David and Rick, he was also drawn to the challenge of Uluru, and climbed it two years after the operation.

Ethan wanted to recover faster and thought that a trip to Bali would prove to him how well he was. At home he had extended himself cautiously, noting that he walked a little further as the days went by. His wife said that he put extra effort into recovering, and did exactly what was called for in the exercise classes. A small test on the boat gangplank showed him that he was normal again.

"I had to get out and stretch for a walk. One hundred yards the first day; next day a little further and so on. Progress was pretty rapid. It depends on the encouragement you get from your spouse. But I was determined to go on this trip. We thoroughly enjoyed it. Swimming, and all activities except that I was slightly thinner than normal. At one point we had to go down a steep gangplank from the ship. Some passengers found it difficult but I could get up and down without any trouble. I was virtually normal."

Barbara's challenge was to find the signs of getting better. She studied her medical past carefully, and identified details that might have contributed to her heart disease.

"After the operation every day for six months I went through in my mind what had led up to it, and how each day I was recovering. I remembered the signs. When I had to hurry or get in to start the car, I could hear the blood rushing and each heartbeat, and the car engine absolutely booming. Never heard that since the operation. After the operation I stood up in front of the mirror to do my hair and said, 'I've got pink lips again!' I had had blue lips, and I hadn't noticed it developing. Pink lips, wow!"

Catherine concentrated on housekeeping tasks to challenge her, and show how well she was. Her challenge was to become self-sufficient as soon as possible.

"After two weeks with each daughter I went back home. I worked to find ways of doing things. I got the vacuum cleaner to see if it was too heavy to lift. I had to find how to open the old garage door without putting too much strain on my muscles. I did that. I had help from the local community services. I don't need anything now. I am completely self-sufficient."

Hank was on a business trip in the USA when he tested himself. And he went surfing, rode a big wave and got his confidence back.

"The operation does knock your confidence. Went to America that September, and I really felt confident and pleased with myself. I don't think I looked at it as a test when I went, but when I got back, I thought that I'd really tested myself. We were in this small boat, fishing sixty miles off the Mexico shore, and the guy I was with had a stent put in a year earlier. I came back thinking to myself, 'I'm all right now.' Quite a psychological boost that trip gave me. Another thing was when I was home surfing alone, and there was one particular wave I caught that was a real high for me. It was probably one of the best waves I've caught ever. I remember it clearly. There was hardly anyone else out there."

Attitude to recovery rate

Erik has a heart specialist he likes very much: 'He sits with you and doesn't talk above you, he asks you questions and you can ask him questions.' This specialist put him in hospital to be given a new drug to strengthen his heart muscle. But, feeling that over the last five years he had recovered sufficiently, Erik had some doubts about the treatment.

"The drug will give a longer function to the heart muscle. He reckons I'm very fit, and he wants to keep me fit. I said, 'Doctor, I'm not that young, I've got good quality out of what life I had. Part of my family perished in Auschwitz, and what I've got is a great bonus. I believe in quality, I don't want to live just for the sake of hanging around.' But this treatment required hospitalisation, because he administers a small dose of the drug at a time, and they can see the reaction immediately. It either works or it doesn't work. You can get heart failure from it. So you've got to be treated in hospital. I'm now on the full dose of it, so maybe he's right. So far so good."

Impatient about his slow rate of recovery, Peter felt his criteria for recovery were not being met. His wife noted that he used to sleep all the time before the operation, and now she saw he had more energy, did more, and was able to keep going longer.

"As far as I'm concerned my body is meant to do certain things, and it had better do them. Why doesn't it get better faster? That is the point. They fixed my heart and it should be right. I'm intolerant of inefficiencies in my body. I was not distressed at not getting better faster, just impatient."

Informants compared their rate of recovery with that of other people who had had the same operation. Chris, who now suffers severe complications, had an 83-year-old friend who recovered much faster. James's recovery ten years ago seemed slower than the recovery of today's patients; yet his close friend's recovery was so fast that it annoyed the family.

"It took me two years from 1989. I don't quite know why. But it's just a huge assault on your body. Recovery seems to be shorter now with people I've talked to. Some people, because they get their heart repaired, get a new burst of life. My friend had his heart operation, and in a few weeks he got an incredible amount of energy he never had before because he was getting a bigger blood supply. His wife said, 'I think I liked him better before he had the operation.' I wasn't like that. I don't know why."

Like James, Ethan had his operation ten years ago. At the time he thought his recovery was quick. But later his rate of recovery changed character.

"You've got the ageing process to go through. Ten years is the usual time a bypass lasts. So now I've got to be careful. I went to a film and my wife parked the car on a hill behind the cinema, and I had difficulty with a walk uphill. Angina. I have to stop, rest and wait for a while. Apart from that I am in reasonable shape."

Catherine monitored the rate at which she recovered, and brought it under control by changing her activities and lowering her expectations.

"I've paced myself all along to make sure that what I do I can handle. And I think that's got me back quicker than anything to recovery. I didn't expect too much, but I didn't sit around waiting for things to happen. It's tremendous not having angina. I don't think I need any more recovery. I garden three hours twice a week for friends ... It's sort of a hobby. I haven't got my own garden, so I do other people's gardens, because I like gardening and to be active."

Two weeks after the operation, Rick went to see his surgeon, and was congratulated on the rate at which he had recovered. His heart was strong, his health was good, and if he were to die unexpectedly, then it would be shown that heart disease was not the cause. He was overjoyed at the success of a new technique that his surgeon tried, and congratulated himself on how he had dropped unhealthy habits.

"Fourteen days after the operation I saw the surgeon and he said, 'Boy, have we done a good job for you!' ... If I did the right things, I would have no problems with my heart. If I was to die in other circumstances, it would show that there was no damage to the heart. That made me feel privileged as well. I have possibly another twenty years or so. I was smart enough—and keen enough to get superfit, to change all those bad smoking and dietary things I used to do."

Barbara felt she recovered rapidly, but was disappointed that the pain stayed with her for so long. The short stay at her golf club before settling in at home seemed helpful.

"Getting better wasn't held up, but the length of the time of the pain was disappointing. I just accepted it. The fact that I had those few days relaxing at the golf club gave me a good start. I was aware after a big surgery you don't pick up quickly. But I was able to cope with daily activities after the golf club stay. We had one more meal brought to us at home. After that I was doing the cooking. As before I had help in the house, washing, and a house cleaner came."

Three years have passed since David's operation, and he seems pleased with his health, comparing it favourably to his life before his unexpected operation and joining his friends in healthy activities, but, even so, he worries about what might happen.

"I was fit beforehand. I weigh 86 kilos now. When I played football I weighed 85 kilos. In the hospital I think I got down to 83 kilos. Then I went back to 86. So it didn't really change my shape or life, or anything. I'm still on Zocor. My cholesterol was 3.2 the last time they took it. The cardiologist doesn't want to see me any more. Am I a time bomb or am I all right?"

Advice to others

Informants wanted to give advice to those who were contemplating heart surgery. They have no technical knowledge to offer, so they say it is important to find medical staff, doctors, cardiac physicians and surgeons who can selectively describe and explain clearly what the operation involves. Seek information, but not too much. It's a gruesome business to ordinary people, as a visit to a surgical intensive care unit will show you. A doctor who can communicate easily, with an understanding of how it feels to be a patient, is of greater benefit to your recovery than someone who imparts just the technical details of the operation itself.

As a patient, there are some things you might be able to do in preparation for the operation. Be as healthy and as fit as you can; quit smoking, eat properly, and if possible exercise to raise your muscle tone and strength. Talk with others who have had the operation. They might have useful tips. Decide on whether you want to recover in a private or public hospital. Have medical insurance, if that is possible. After the operation, accept the pain for a few days, and the fact that natural fear is normal. After all, it's an operation for your life. The fear of surgery will dissipate when you see that first you have no alternative, second the operation is remarkably successful, and third recovery is rapid. A positive approach will help add years of comfort to your life. Afterwards, if you fully accept your ageing body, you can benefit greatly from learning new skills, and planning within manageable limits modest tests to challenge and evaluate and extend your recovery. Recently, Lachlan, who had retired from university, became a graphic artist, did much writing, and a lot of reading, learned to use a lathe, and now makes furniture. From this he concludes that the best advice he can give is to keep mentally and physically alert in recovery and retirement.

"I have both a physical and a mental life which is very active. For those recovering from a bypass, my advice would always be if you feel that you haven't recovered so well then get active mentally *and* physically."

Erik had no direct advice to give, but he knew, deeply, what had helped him.

"I'll tell you what I felt helped me a lot. I'm lucky, I've got a doctor who came to my bedside with a model of a heart, explained exactly to me what is likely to happen and he treated me like somebody who's not totally ignorant. I can listen to somebody who is expert and understand what he tells me. That made me feel more confident. I go to him now once every three or four months, he sits with me, and takes three-quarters of an hour. At the end he types a little letter explaining things to me in writing, with the details of the drugs he wants me to take. When I walk out I feel confident. I like to know what I'm doing."

James was adamant that he would recommend the public over the private hospital system on grounds of technical competence. Also, the prospective patient needs to feel assured his surgeon is competent.

"I would absolutely recommend a *public* hospital. At mine the professorial unit assembled two cardiac emergency teams at the same time. There was nowhere else you could possibly do that. I've got private health cover now, but I would say to go to the public hospital I went to. The success rate's extremely good now. Knowing that you've got a good surgeon is important, and that he's done lots of operations."

Unlike James, Liam advised that you should go to the private hospital that had cared for him, and suggested that not all others were up to an adequate standard.

"Go to the private hospital I went to. We have a cardiac club; we all wear the red badge of courage."

David recommended that patients should not push themselves too hard; and they should agree to the operation because it is such a success.

"People who have high cholesterol shouldn't exert themselves. If you've got a medical or a health problem, have it with your *heart*. They can fix your heart. I am very thankful my problem was *heart* and not cancer or another disease. I have a friend who has just been diagnosed with Parkinson's. It's devastating for him, for his family, for everyone. But my problem, I think, is fixed; but his problem is just starting. I haven't had any complications. Friends of mine who've had it done are virtually in the same boat as me."

Brad had very little to do with organisations or support groups such as the local heart association and thought a good counsellor, or a person who'd been through the experience, would be the best to give advice. For himself he anticipated returning to golf, or perhaps taking up something that was entirely new to ensure he maintained self-confidence.

"The best advice is to feel that you're doing well, and that you're still worthwhile. Make sure you haven't lost it, totally. Accept that you lost some of what you had, but you could still be a vibrant person. It's a matter of having something to feel satisfied about, and to be looking forward to. One problem with going back to golf is that you're not going to be playing as well as before. It may be best to dice that totally, and get stuck into woodwork. Anything you do is going to be good if it's new. I think there's a lot in that. I would like to try to get back to golf. How the heart would go now I'm not too sure, but it shouldn't be too bad. Could try the par three golf course first, with a golf buggy."

Catherine advised that you should learn as much as you need to know about the operation itself—avoiding the technical details—and be prepared well for the *early* stages of recovery. All this was given to her by her surgeon.

"The more information you have about the actual job, what it entails, the better. The surgeon explained everything to me, what he would do, how he would do it. But I don't think you need to have too much knowledge about the *nasty* parts of it. I think you need to know that for a while at first it is going to be unpleasant."

Chris regrets not having gone to the local doctor at the first sign of heart attack when he was working on his boat.

"If you think you are having a heart attack, or having something so unusual you have never experienced it before, don't delay like I did. If I had gone to the local doctor four years ago, the permanent damage to the heart that I now have would probably be far less. If I hadn't been so stubborn working on the boat, had gone after the first episode, there would have been less damage. About 35 per cent is damaged. Dead, just not working."

Peter advised visiting the intensive care unit to know what the immediate result of the operation appears to be.

"One of the things they really want you to do is go and look at the recovery room, which has got all these dials and instruments and recording apparatus. So you don't have a horrible fright when you come to."

Lachlan believed that fear of not recovering in hospital is a cause of slow recovery among some patients, and recommends the use of entertainment to distract the patient from the fears associated with the operation.

"I had a wonderful tape on a Walkman that helped me to recover in hospital, Garrison Keillor's *Lake Wobegon Days*, a selection of autumn, summer, winter, spring. Wonderful to be lying in bed laughing my head off. It's no use advising people about recovery. They must *want* to do it."

Rick advised a similar positive attitude of mind for the recovery, but based his advice on his sporting experiences.

"My local doctor said that I was a walking symbol of what can be done through surgery. Whether it's come from your sporting background or whatever, there's the positive mental attitude to succeed and the willingness to get physically fit. And the discipline."

Hank advised that you should get yourself health insurance. Years after the operation he needed a stent inserted into a blocked blood vessel, and because he was insured he could decide when that would be done, rather than wait, as many uninsured patients must.

"I rang the surgeon and said, 'Hey, I want the stent.' He said, 'Okay, I'll do you this week.' Because I was insured I could be done immediately. It cost the insurance company thousands. When I wasn't insured, years ago, it cost nothing! But then I ran a pretty good chance of not getting done in time."

(12)

Later discomfort and problems

The heart bypass operation has a high success rate, and most patients no longer suffer badly from heart disease. But however successful the operation and however gratifying the recovery, there is always the chance that serious complications or minor problems can arise.

Minor problems occur if you get a cold soon after the operation; you could panic a little about the thought of living alone and need pain-killers for longer than expected; walking at home might be difficult and stressful; you might be too impatient and want to advance the rate of recovery beyond what your body can accept.

Serious complications centring on the heart's functioning may arise. The informants' experiences points clearly to one fact: after heart bypass surgery it is essential to notify your doctor of anything that you suspect might be affecting the operation of your heart.

Hank—'These grafts don't always work'

Hank was told that when he had had a heart attack, part of his heart muscle had died because on the left-hand side of his heart an artery which pumped blood to his body had become blocked. The surgeon used a mammary artery to take the blood flow around the blockage. At the time it was evident that another artery was also blocked.

"The other one—on the heart's right-hand side—is a smaller artery, and that just pumps the blood to your lungs to get oxygenated. They bypassed that one too with another piece of mammary artery. That was the minor thing. They thought, 'Well, we may as well do it, because we've cut him open anyway.'"

During his recovery, Hank had pains that lasted for three years.

"Three years almost to the day after the operation, I was at work, and I had pains in the chest. I'd been having them ever since, on and off. Everyone had been saying, 'Stop worrying.' My wife kept saying, 'You're fixed. Stop complaining. You're fine. I'm the one you should be worrying about.'"

During those three years Hank had been seeing his specialist regularly and was told that he was healthy. But one day a woman in Hank's office at work thought he looked ill and should go to hospital. There he was told the second graft had not been successful.

"All the time the specialist is telling me that I'm fine, putting me on his exercise bikes, and saying, 'You're meant to do 60 per cent and I had you on 90 per cent. You're fine.' Then the woman in the office noticed I was still having pains—she's very conscious of keeping me alive—so I went to the local hospital ... I end up in the ambulance, going to the *city* hospital and they give me an angiogram, and they say, 'Hey, the secondary bypass blocked. It's not working.' I ask why, and their best answer was, 'Shit happens!' I say, 'I can get an answer like that down at the hotel! Can't you be more specific?' And they say, 'No. There's a chance that these grafts don't always work. And yours is not working.' I ask, 'Aren't there any guarantees?' And they say, 'No. Not really.' So I'm thinking, 'Well, I *knew* I was getting pains.'"

What was he to do? By this time Hank had taken out family health insurance and had a choice as to where he would be hospitalised.

"We'd only let the health insurance lapse because of the school fees. So now I've got health insurance cover at the city hospital, and I've got this beautiful room, lovely view of the sports grounds and over the city. They are saying, 'You're not going to die. Either we can give you an angioplasty now, or you can go home and think about it. Ring up and book in. The surgeon's going for his holiday the week after next.' So the surgeon asks, 'What are you going to do?' I say, 'I want to go home.'"

Hank was taken home, but when he got there he reconsidered his position.

"I began to think to myself, 'You idiot. You *should've* done it then and there.' I rang up and said, 'I want this thing done.' They said, 'Come in the following Thursday.' I turned up, they gave me an angioplasty on the Friday ... I've been fine ever since. Since I've had the stent, I can feel it. Just a little. I would say I haven't had any problems at all. But last week, when I was in Tokyo, I had a bit of an episode."

Hank's specialist gave him more tests that seemed from Hank's view to be related to his heart's performance under stress.

"While I was there I said to the specialist that I had these bad feelings last week. He said, 'If you ever have them again, sit down.'"

Brad—a second bypass operation

Within two months of his 1981 bypass operation Brad had the original symptoms return, this time with little pain. Deeply disappointed, he saw his surgeon and cardiologist, who prescribed medication. He is still taking it today. Brad believes that one of the bypassed arteries blocked immediately after the operation.

Altogether Brad counted eighteen different medications prescribed for him. The medication not only controlled the original cool feeling in his throat, but also produced frequent headaches or depression. Brad reduced his time at work and his activities at home. In 1989 he had another heart attack; it did little damage. A second and third heart attack were worse, with congestion, deep pain, and much sweating. Following an angiogram early in 1990 he had a second bypass operation. In the second hospital he found the medical staff were not as competent; their manner, caring, and mode of communication were poor. Preparation for the operation seemed less elaborate—little shaving, no pre-operation body washing routines—and he saw less of the anaesthetist. He had more trouble breathing, the respirator tube was in his throat longer. But this time someone was there to help him wake up in ICU. Although he didn't feel confident about the results of the second operation, it was successful.

Chris— 'He said I had an arrhythmia problem'

Chris had two serious episodes that have affected him ever since his bypass operation. Late in 1998, two months after the operation, he fainted for about a half a minute. He treated the episode as a minor event, and decided against calling his cardiologist. A month later he had a similar experience, but this time in far more threatening circumstances.

"Four or five weeks later I was listening to music until midnight. I got up, turned off the equipment, went down on one knee and put my hand on the lamp switch to turn it off. All of sudden, I couldn't do anything with my hand. I didn't know whether I needed to press the switch, or flick it, or what to do. I passed out. Fell on the floor, nearly pulled a massive amplifier down on my head. Could have killed me. Unconscious. Don't know how long. I came to, in a pile of wire, looking up at the amplifier teetering over me, with the lamp shining six inches from my eyes. Next day we made an emergency appointment with the cardiologist."

The cardiologist said Chris should have phoned her immediately after the *first* episode and gone directly to hospital. He was sent to a specialist for a complete test. It appeared to be worthless.

"Zero! Nothing showed up on the tests at all. Later the cardiologist could not explain why the two episodes occurred, and said, 'There are so many things about hearts that we don't know. Next you go for a day procedure with a cardiologist who specialises in heart rhythm.' My cardiologist describes herself as a plumber, and she said this man was an electrician. The procedure involved being anaesthetised, and then, as it beats, the heart is put under an increasing rate of pressure. Towards the end of the procedure he explained that all sorts of things can go wrong during the test. So he had two anaesthetists ready, and an assistant. All the latest gear too. It was done, and then my heart stopped and they had to resuscitate me. He said that I had an arrhythmia problem, and that was probably the cause of the fainting episodes. My heart suddenly beat at a drastically reduced rate, blood flow to my head was immediately cut off, and I went down."

What is the answer to arrhythmia? He was told it was serious, possibly fatal, and that the recommended treatment was effective, but the reason was not securely known.

"'First, it is a serious problem,' the specialist said. 'If you go into arrhythmia again, you'll probably be dead in four minutes.' Treatment is by medication, Aratac, where you start with a substantial dose and you reduce it as much as possible. The specialist said, 'No one knows why it controls arrhythmia. Clinical observation shows it works with some and not others, but we don't

know why. We'll try that first.' He said the drawbacks to the treatment are
that the Aratac has an adverse long-term effect on the liver and intestines,
and for that reason was not prescribed for more than three years."

The specialist also said that if the drug failed to work, he would
recommend inserting a defibrillator inside the chest behind the
ribs. Because Chris was so slim the defibrillator would be uncomfortable. He might not be able to lie on his preferred side in bed,
and might have to make special arrangements for placement of his
car seatbelt because it would go exactly where the device is fixed.
Also, serious psychological problems can arise in some patients.

"Next thing is to have a defibrillator fitted. Size of an audio cassette. It
gives you an immediate impulse that corrects the heart's actions and
restores the heartbeat. Some patients are unable to live with the defibrillator inside them because all day they are thinking, 'When is it going to go
off? Am I going to get a shock? When's it going to work?' It becomes a psychological problem, and they come back and say, 'Please, take it out. I can't
stand it.' And the specialist said there is pain and discomfort associated
with it. The other thing is a risk of infection—not an inconsiderable risk—
and there is always a risk later of the body rejecting the defibrillator. Then
it would be taken out. 'What then?' I asked. 'You're back on Aratac.'"

Chris had to make up his mind as to what treatment he wanted.
His specialist advised him to look at the defibrillator as an insurance
policy—that is, it may never work, but if it did his life would be saved.

"That's pretty dramatic stuff! He added, 'Hopefully a slightly smaller defibrillator version will be available soon that would not be so uncomfortable for
you. Go away, think about it. But don't think about it for too long.' I've been
thinking about it since late 1998. Too long. I can't stay in sunshine. I haven't
been able to wear a short-sleeved shirt because of skin sensitivity to ultraviolet sunlight, another side effect of the Aratac. It makes my life intolerable.
You wouldn't want to go outside at all. Anyway its up to me to make up my
mind. I go back to see him soon. I'll ask the cardiologist for her opinion
again. I'll review the situation. And if I can drive myself to make up my mind
I'll have this defibrillator fitted. I asked whether or not I should be driving.
'No!' he said, and I said that I had a lovely car, I like to drive. He said, 'You
never know when it's going to happen. You'll get no warning. You'll be there
one moment, and you'll be gone the next.' So the drama hasn't ended yet."

Liam—'There's clogging at either end of the vein bypass'

Liam felt well until about six years after his operation. He learned that research showed that in some cases putting in veins where once there had been arteries is not effective in the long term. Veins do not have the same muscle layer as arteries, are not as elastic, and do not conduct the blood as efficiently especially when scar tissue forms at the point where the vein is grafted on to the artery to by-pass original blockages. Plaque can build up. So some patients have to go through the operation again.

> "I've had a bit of a problem for six years. I started to get pain, and an angiogram showed I was having a bit of clogging at either end of the vein bypass. The artery bypass was okay, and diet must have been effective for the lesser clogged artery. It hadn't changed. So I had the angioplasty, in April 1993, and that relieved the pain. That often happens. It's a minimal procedure and you're out next day. The procedure pushes the blood vessel out, but it doesn't keep it out. So about four years later I started to get pains again. In the meantime they had developed stents ... They put one in, then another in after the other. Three stents stayed okay and held open the vein graft."

Lachlan—ten years after the first bypass ...

In November 1995, ten years after his first bypass operation, Lachlan felt strangely ill after climbing a mountain. In 1996 he was walking up an incline on a golf links and found that he couldn't make it. He saw his cardiologist, who told him that after his bypass operation four vein grafts had blocked while one artery bypass was still functioning well. He was taken to hospital and stabilised with an angiogram patch, so no operation was needed.

But he discovered from other patients that if you have a vein graft, you may need a second operation between seven and fifteen years later, depending on your body and lifestyle.

He soon had another episode, and, thinking it was a heart attack, he went back to hospital. He was in need of a *second* operation. The surgeon assured him the risk factor was about one per cent.

This time he had an artery removed from his arm, and early the next morning had an eight-hour operation.

He compared experiences of the 1995 operation with those of 1985. He felt the same sense of being choked by the respirator tube. On the second occasion the nurse gave him paper and pencil; he wrote her a coherent message but she could not read it because, being unable to see his writing, he had printed each letter on top of the last. The mirror showed he had a 40 per cent larger face. Also this time his lung was partly collapsed, and it was painful when a pressure mask was forced over his face to help expand his collapsed lung. He remembered having a morphine-induced dream after the second operation; also he entertained himself reading many books during his recovery in a private room. This time he attended rehabilitation exercise classes. There, from lifting weights to strengthen his muscles, a shoulder that had been damaged during the operation froze stiff and had to be treated separately. Now he feels fully recovered from the second operation.

"Of all the major operations, the bypass is the most known about, and the least to fear. I am perfectly recovered except for one wrist that's a little less strong than it was."

Kim—'You've had a stroke'

After his operation in July 1997, Kim had been well until he experienced an unusual slurring in his speech.

"Two months later ... in the morning I was home having cornflakes, sitting at the dining-room table and my wife came down, and she asked, 'How do you feel?' and I said, 'All right.' She came over and said I had dribbled down my chin, and I'm *fastidious* about eating. I *never* dribble. She said my mouth was down, my eye was down, my whole face was down on one side. She put her arms round me and she said, 'Darling, you've had a stroke.' I can remember, because I knew when she asked, 'How do you feel?' I couldn't say what I wanted to say. My brain knew the words, just couldn't bring them out. She rang the hospital, and they arrived five minutes later, but I'm going a-hundred-miles-an-hour by this time. No problem at all. They were bringing in the stretcher, and I said, 'Don't worry, I'll walk out with you.' I get up. At this stage I'm not slurring words. I walk out, hop in the ambulance, down to the casualty ward. Immediately you feel a bit crook when you get into a casualty environment because there's sick people moaning and groaning all around.

They say, 'We're going to give you the CT scan.' It showed part of a clot had gone through my brain and had affected me. Still has affected me in terms of being able to hold an erection. I can still have sex and all the rest of it, but it's a lot more difficult than a normal guy would have. So I had to stay in hospital for six days. I felt terrific. By 3 o'clock that afternoon I didn't know I had a stroke. Been back to work for two weeks in the middle of that period, and, touch wood, only once since then I've felt crook, and that was self-inflicted. So then I went to the surgeon from September '97 when I had that stroke through February '98, and he adjusted various medications. I take them last thing before bed at night. Whack my pills down. I've never been back to him since February last year and I'm supposed to go every three months. Now that's stupidity on my side, and different friends of mine—two are doctors—keep saying I should go. I say I feel terrific! But I must go back just to show him that the reason I haven't been back is because I'm looking good. He probably thinks I've died."

Less than three months later, Kim died aged 60. More than four hundred people attended his funeral.

$$\textbf{(13)}$$

Conclusions and recommendations

The informants' experiences show the signs of heart disease vary from one person to another, and often seem like private discomforts, minor illnesses or passing incapacities. Sometimes the signs are dramatic and painful, at other times hardly noticeable or irritating, and simply a little unusual.

This experience indicates that you should not attempt to diagnose heart trouble yourself: don't ignore the unusual signs of something wrong, don't assume that minor complaints will simply go away, and never feel your doctor will be bothered or irritated when you present with complaints that you have decided might be trivial.

To find out the basic signs of heart trouble, seek expert information that you can understand and relate it to yourself, ask for help from a doctor, and get brochures from your national heart authority. And if you're over 50, and your family members have had heart trouble, keep up-to-date on information about heart disease and its causes.

One cause of your heart disease could have been due to your not seeking expert medical advice early. If your heart beats very fast or chaotically, or if your chest is in pain, and it spreads up your throat and into your arms, seek medical help immediately. You might be having a heart attack.

The causes of heart attack and heart disease are not fully known, and much is still to be discovered about the heart. However, your national heart authority makes what is securely known available regularly and updates important new material clearly. Keep well informed about heart trouble and how it relates to you, especially if you're at risk of heart disease.

Your doctor can advise you on the risk of heart disease in your case: the doctor will need to know your family medical history, levels of cholesterol in your blood, your smoking habits, and your diet, blood pressure, weight, and exercise habits. The doctor can tell you exactly what to do to lower the risks, and what risks you cannot control at all. It costs nothing to be well informed and clearly advised, and the benefits to you and those close to you are enormous.

People with heart disease accept they have no authority in the decision to operate on their heart. This is a life-and-death decision, and it is usually made *for* you, not *by* you. You will probably need to feel confident about the surgeon who acts on the decision and takes you through a bypass operation. You will need to trust the surgeon's competence and personal skills.

If you have time, you can find out about the competence of various surgeons. Many people do not have the time. And what would those who do have time want to know? The reputation, personal qualities and interpersonal style are what patients seem to use when they judge their surgeons. You could ask around about the surgeon's reputation. Some people do. Others accept their cardiologist's recommended surgeon as the best that they can get.

Informants showed something of the trust they want to feel in a surgeon. The feeling of trust was established when they asked the surgeon questions to help understand both the technical aspects of the operation and the recovery afterwards. From their experiences it appears that you will feel confident about the surgeon when you understand enough about your heart trouble and the operations they will do for you. To help you manage the natural anxiety you feel about the risk of death, pain and complications, seek as full an account of the surgeon's task as you can tolerate.

How full will that account be? Your surgeon will hesitate to give you a complete professional and technical story of the work to be done on your diseased heart. Surgeons feel and know that telling *all* the details might worry the patient; also, telling too little might be anxiety-provoking. They make a professional decision based on what they know of you, and then give an account with the detail they feel you want. How can you help them reach that point? You can help the surgeon by setting a limit on what you need to know by simply withdrawing your interest in detailed surgical procedures. To reach this point with your surgeon, listen carefully to what is being said or shown to you, and state your feelings clearly about what has been done and said. The surgeon's understanding of you will be enhanced, and you will be well informed about their work, and in time your curiosity will rest. Your feeling of trust for the surgeon will be established, and you will anticipate going with the surgeon's flow of work and expectations for you.

Your cardiologist's choice of surgeon is your best initial advice; your trust in the surgeon will come from how attentively you listen to what the surgeon says, doesn't say, and will not say without your questions. By this stage you and your surgeon will be working together on your heart, and you will start becoming a patient in hospital.

Once you are in hospital, you'll be overwhelmed by the work of becoming a patient. For a day or so you are an object without much control of your activities. Your task is to sit and accept the flow of work around you and be the patient. You can handle your natural fear of death in many ways. One well-known way is to consider the alternative to a bypass operation.

After the operation you will feel fairly battered. But you will be the centre of attention, and no matter what pain or discomfort you feel, things can only get better. This attitude is strongly recommended by other patients, and seems to be a great help to medical staff. It will help you to accept drugs for the pain that you cannot control, and help you to dispense with those drugs when you feel your recovery falling back under your control.

As a rule, you can expect to recover from the operation as most other people do. But because complete knowledge about the heart is yet to be found, complications may occur during the operation, in your early recovery, or in the longer term. Complications are part of the riskiness of pursuing good health through surgery, and medical help is always available to manage any complications. If you feel bad after you and the surgeon have done what you can to recover from the operation, then seek help immediately.

Normal recovery leads to changes in lifestyle. Your diet will change; you will exercise more systematically; perhaps you will learn much about recovery from fellow-patients as well as staff in the rehabilitation classes at the hospital or after your hospital stay. Unusual and unexpected experiences in recovery should be brought immediately to the attention of your doctor or cardiologist.

People vary in their rate and methods of recovery. For example, it takes between six and eight weeks for the chest to heal. This will affect your use of a car as a passenger or a driver. There will be limits put on your return to work and use of heavy effort. Questions about lifting, sports, bathing, having sex, going to work, home chores, using cars or bicycles, and sleep problems are readily answered by your doctor. As a rule moderation will be suggested, and the idea that you ought to recover at your own rate will be recommended.

In principle you decide on your recovery rate; but if you decide not to follow medical and para-medical advice, others might be victims of that decision, and resent it. Medical advice is given not for you alone; it is also for those who care for you.

Some people want to know how their recovery is going. To find out, consider giving yourself a graded series of tests: find a serious challenge, and compare yourself with others and their achievements. If you want to test yourself, do so with others.

Basic interest in routine daily activities can change. Your interest in food can go and your sense of taste can disappear, speech and hearing can be affected, concentration on details can go, and your vision can falter. Your doctor will probably advise you to wait a little and be patient; if problems like these continue, seek medical advice again.

Your image of yourself might change. Some people feel depressed at having lost the identity they once had. Others find themselves more vulnerable to threats; a few enlarge threats they once would easily have managed. Depression and anxiety after an operation are common and not difficult to manage for most people. Often people are not aware of their depression, and many dismisses it as a character weakness, or temporary tiredness, while some develop an uncharacteristic dependency on those who care for them.

The fear of being vulnerable and a fall in your self-worth usually pass with plans to go on a vacation, a decision to take up new skills, a clear awareness of getting better, and the decision to limit your approach to work. If worries and depression continue, seek further help from your doctor, a psychologist, a personal counsellor, or a psychiatrist.

Finally, people who are ill often learn from one another. So if you are to have a bypass operation and have the time, find out what other people did, felt and thought. How did they prepare themselves physically? What did they ask their doctors? What goes on in the intensive care unit? What is it like waking up after an operation? How soon can you use the bathroom alone? What kind of exercises help you to recover? How long were they away from work? Did it change their life? How? Answers to these questions can help you become a capable patient and enhance the natural progress of your recovery. The reward for knowing how to be a capable patient will be a longer life and the freedom to live comfortably without heart trouble.

Glossary

anaesthesia

a loss of feeling or sensation in part or all of your body due to injury or disease of a nerve. Usually the term is applied to the reduction in or abolition of a person's sense of pain before surgery.

angina, angina attack

a sense of suffocation or suffocating pain

angina pectoris

pain in the middle of the chest brought about by exercise and eased with rest. It may spread to your jaws and arms. It happens when the heart's demand for blood exceeds the supply of the coronary arteries. Usually it is due to coronary artery atheroma, i.e. degeneration of the artery walls either by scarring or building up of plaque. It may be treated with drugs; when they are not effective a coronary angioplasty or coronary bypass may be appropriate.

Anginine

a nitrate tablet you place under the tongue or chew. The tablet will rapidly relieve anginal chest pain.

angiography, angiogram

the X-ray examination of blood vessels. A dye, opaque to X-rays, is injected into the artery, and a rapid X-ray film is taken. The results indicate where arteries are narrowing and preventing an adequate supply of blood reaching its goal.

angioplasty

involves the repair by surgery of an obstructed or narrowed artery. *See also* coronary angioplasty.

aortic valve

a valve in the heart between the left ventricle and the aorta, the main artery of the body. The valve stops blood from returning to the ventricle from the aorta.

Aratac

a prescribed drug used to treat cardiac arrhythmias.

arrhythmia

deviation from the normal sinus rhythm of the beating heart. In the wall of the right atrium of the heart lies the natural pacemaker of the heart, and it controls the rhythm of the whole heart by way of the autonomic nervous system (ANS). The ANS produces electrical impulses that spread through the heart and cause it to contract normally. When the normal production or spreading of these impulses is disturbed the heartbeats may become arrhythmical. The symptoms of arrhythmia are palpitations, breathlessness, and chest pain. In serious cases the heart may stop. The cause of arrhythmia is heart disease, but it can occur without warning or apparent cause.

arteries

the blood vessels that carry the blood away from the heart. All but the pulmonary artery carry oxygenated blood to nourish the body's vital organs. Artery walls are made of smooth muscle fibre which contracts and relaxes under the control of the sympathetic nervous system.

arteriosclerosis

a term often used to mean atherosclerosis, and referring to a process in which the walls of the small arteries become thick due to hypertension or simply ageing.

aspirin

a drug used widely to relieve pain, inflammation and fever, headache, toothache, and other discomforts.

atherosclerosis

a disease of the arteries in which fatty plaques grow and adhere to the inside of the artery wall and impede adequate blood flow.

atrium

refers to either of the two upper chambers of the heart. Their muscular walls are thinner than those of the ventricles: the left atrium gets oxygenated blood from the lungs via the pulmonary vein, while the right atrium receives deoxygenated blood from the venae cavae.

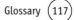

autologous blood supply

a donation of blood to a blood bank which, in turn, makes it available to you at the time of your operation. This procedure reduces the likelihood of blood infection.

blood pressure

the pressure of blood against walls of the main arteries. The pressure is high when the heart's ventricles contract and lowest when they relax and are refilling. Blood pressure is measured in millimetres of mercury at that point in the arm where the pressure is similar to that of blood leaving the heart. In a normal young adult, the highest pressure when ventricles are contracting would be about 120 mm, and the lowest about 80 mm when the ventricles are relaxing, i.e. 120/80. Individuals differ in blood pressure due to many factors other than physical health and heredity, e.g. emotional states such as fear, excitement, or stress, or to muscular efforts.

bypass

see cardiopulmonary bypass and coronary artery bypass graft.

cardiac ward

the hospital ward set aside for the care of patients recovering from treatment for heart disease.

cardiologist

a highly trained medical doctor who has specialised in studies of the structure, function and diseases of the heart.

cardiopulmonary bypass

a method for maintaining the body's circulation when it has been stopped for heart surgery. This is achieved with a heart–lung machine. From the body, blood is taken in tubes which have been put into the venae cavae and sent through the machine; the blood is filled with oxygen and returned to the body under pressure by way of the femoral artery. This allows the surgeon to repair the heart or replace its valves.

cardiopulmonary resuscitation (CPR)

the means by which medical staff aim to prevent the imminent death of a person whose heart has apparently failed and must be restarted. The procedure involves compressing or massaging the chest and mouth-to-mouth breathing.

cholesterol

a vital fatty material in the blood and most body tissue. It is processed largely in the liver, and is normally concentrated in the blood between

3.6 and 7.8 mol./L. Too much cholesterol in the blood is frequently associated with degeneration of artery walls due to fatty plaques forming on them and limiting blood circulation, which might lead to thrombosis. Rich in animal fats, the Western diet may contribute to the role that high cholesterol plays in heart disease.

codeine

a commonly used pain-killer, derived from morphine but less powerful, less toxic and rarely addictive. It is administered by mouth or injection, and has side effects, e.g. constipation, dizziness, drowsiness, nausea, vomiting.

collateral blood vessels

another way provided for blood circulation through secondary blood vessels when the primary vessels are blocked. Also communication channels between the blood vessels that supply the heart.

coronary angioplasty

a means by which the narrowed part of a coronary artery is stretched by the inflation of a balloon brought into the artery at the tip of a flexible catheter. When the balloon is inflated the flow of blood in the artery is improved.

coronary arteries

arteries that supply blood to the heart. From the aorta (the main artery of the body) come the right and left arteries, just above the aortic valve, and they branch around the heart.

coronary artery bypass graft

a surgeon's procedure for enriching blood in a badly nourished heart muscle by transplanting an expendable vein/artery around areas of atherosclerotic narrowing. The grafted vein/artery bypasses the blockage in the heart's artery.

coronary heart disease

disease of the arteries that branch around the heart occurs when the arteries become no longer able to provide adequate blood to the heart muscle. One main cause is an excessive narrowing of the coronary arteries that impedes blood flow. This may be followed by myocardial infarction—death of a part of the heart muscle—which provokes the experience of a 'heart attack'.

coronary occlusion

the closing or obstruction of coronary arteries.

deep vein thrombosis (DVT)

after an operation blood clots may establish themselves in the deep veins of the calf and thigh where they cannot be easily seen. It is thought that DVT can be prevented by the wearing of elastic stockings that go from hip to toe, or halfway down both legs.

defibrillator

an apparatus that administers a controlled electric shock to return the heart to its normal rhythm. It may be used when the heart has stopped because of ventricular fibrillation, i.e. when many muscle fibres of the heart begin to beat chaotically and quickly, thus making it impossible for the heart to work in a synchronised and systematic way. The apparatus involves placing electrodes on the chest over the heart, or directly to the heart after chest surgery. It is possible to insert a small device into or near the chest close to the heart to start the heart running normally if chaotic beats begin.

diabetes mellitus

a disorder in which the body's sugars are not oxidised to produce energy because of a poor supply of the pancreatic hormone, insulin. This accumulation of sugar appears in the blood and then the urine, and the sufferer becomes excessively thirsty, loses weight, and must urinate very often. The disorder can be inherited, and also may arise after stress. The disease appears to be of two types; it may even arise in childhood. It is becoming more common and requires close medical attention and special treatment.

ectopic beats or heartbeats

heartbeats caused by some impulse generated from outside the normal source. Usually they are unexpected in timing, and may occur because of any form of heart disease, or from nicotine due to smoking or caffeine from drinking excessive coffee. It is as if your heart misses a beat.

electrocardiogram (ECG)

the recording of electrical activity of the heart on a moving strip of paper. It employs an electrocardiograph that helps in diagnosing heart disease by identifying changes in the ECG.

endorphins

chemical compounds that occur naturally in the brain and have pain-relieving characteristics like those of a drug. They originate from a substance in the pituitary gland.

endotracheal breathing tube

a tube inserted down the throat past the vocal cords into the windpipe and the lungs to assist in breathing after the lungs have been out of operation during heart surgery. It prevents swallowing, speaking and coughing, and feels most uncomfortable. Its removal brings great relief.

haemodialysis

a technique for removing waste or poisons from the blood by using the principle of dialysis. It is used for patients whose kidneys do not function, and the process operates with an artificial kidney or dialyser: blood is taken from an artery, circulated through the dialyser, and returned to the body through a vein.

heart attack

a common term for myocardial infarction, the death of a part of the heart muscle due to an inadequate supply of nourishing blood. As a rule it occurs in the left ventricle. Some symptoms are: sudden severe chest pain; pain spreads to arms and throat; heartbeat rhythm is upset; cardiac arrest. It is best to be taken immediately to a hospital for coronary care. With appropriate treatment, most survivors return to an active and full life.

heart–lung bypass machine

See cardiopulmonary bypass or heart–lung machine.

heart–lung machine

a machine that takes over temporarily from the heart and lungs during a cardiopulmonary bypass. In the machine, a pump keeps up the circulation while another device oxygenates the blood, allowing the surgeon to repair the heart or replace its valves. Sometimes the machine is called a 'washing machine'. *See also* cardiopulmonary bypass.

heart rate

the number of times per minute that the heat pumps; the number of heartbeats in a minute. Normally a healthy heart beats 60 to 100 times per minute.

heparin

a natural anticoagulant that is produced by the liver and in white blood cells, as well as in other places, and which prevents the final stages of blood clotting. In serious cases of blood clotting a purified form of heparin is extracted. Its main side effect is incessant bleeding.

hepatitis

serious liver inflammation caused by viruses, poisons or abnormal conditions in the immune system. It appears in various forms and can be transmitted in various ways.

hypertension

high blood pressure in the arteries. Its cause in a particular case may be unknown; it is often found in association with kidney disease, endocrine diseases, or disease of the arteries. It is without symptoms until the consequences of hypertension are noted. It may be responsible for heart failure, cerebral haemorrhage or kidney failure. In most cases it is treated by long-term drug therapy to lower the blood pressure and keep it within a normal range.

infarct and infarction

infarction is the death of all or part of an organ due to the obstruction in the artery that carries blood to the organ. An infarct is a small localised area of dead tissue produced in this way.

informed consent

your consent to be a patient, given to your surgeon and related personnel, because a surgeon needs legal permission to operate on you. You are expected to sign a form to allow the surgeon to do the operation and be in control of the operation and your recovery, and it is understood that you want all this to be done (your consent) and that you know what you are in for (you are informed). This implies that you trust the surgeon to do the best that can be done no matter what, and that you know what the risks are.

infusionist

the person in charge of the slow injection of drugs, especially pain-killers, into a vein so as to make it possible for your body to endure and recover from surgery.

intensive care unit (ICU, SICU or ITU)

intensive care unit, surgical intensive care unit or intensive therapy unit. A hospital unit where special multidisciplinary staff give intensive care to seriously ill patients or those in need of post-operative technical support after heart or chest operations.

left anterior descending arteries

left main coronary arteries.

mitral valve

a heart valve with two flaps attached to the walls of the opening between the left atrium and the left ventricle. The valve allows the blood to flow from the atrium to the ventricle but not back.

myocardial infarction

a heart attack.

nil orally

a hospital phrase meaning the patient must not be fed until the operation or treatment is over.

Nitrolingual (pumpspray)

glyceryl trinitrate. A treatment for acute angina; can be sprayed under the tongue by the patient.

oesophageal reflux

regurgitation of acid or peptic juices from the stomach due probably to inflammation of the oesophagus (gullet), the muscular tube that extends from the pharynx to the stomach.

Panadol

a commonly used pain-killer.

pericarditis

inflammation of the membranous sac around the heart.

physiotherapist

a person trained in physiotherapy, the branch of treatment that uses physical procedures to promote healing. They are essential to the recovery and rehabilitation of patients who have had surgery. Physio-therapists use light, infra-red and ultraviolet rays, heat, electric current, hydrotherapy, manipulation, massage, stretching and exercises.

pulmonary arteries

two arteries that carry the blood from the heart's right ventricle to each lung; the only arteries that carry deoxygenated blood. Inside the lung each of the arteries divides into fine branches that end in capillaries in the walls of the lungs.

pulmonary embolism

a clot of blood that moves from your leg to your lungs and obstructs the pulmonary artery or one of its branches. If it is large it can produce heart failure or death; if it is small it can cause the death of lung tissue, pleurisy, or coughing of blood.

pulmonary veins

veins that carry oxygenated blood from the lungs to the left atrium where it passes into the left ventricle and by way of the aorta to the arteries that nourish the organs and limbs.

quadruple bypass

a bypass operation in which four bypass grafts are needed to remedy four blockages of the coronary arteries.

saphenous veins

on the leg's surface are two veins that drain blood from the foot. One is short and runs up the back of the calf to join the popliteal vein behind the knee; the other is the longest vein in the body, and runs from the foot, up the inside of the leg to the groin, and joins with the femoral vein.

shunt

a passage that joins two of the body's channels and diverts blood or other fluids from one to another. It is one means by which it is possible to ensure blood flows along an artery that has become blocked.

stent

a tiny splint placed inside a blood vessel to maintain an open space so that blood flow is not severely impeded. It can be inserted by means of a flexible catheter.

systemic arteries

the arteries that carry oxygenated blood from the left side of the heart via the aorta to the limbs and organs of the body.

systemic veins

the veins that carry blood away from vital organs to the right side of the heart and through it to the lungs for oxygenation in the pulmonary arteries.

thrombosis

a condition whereby the blood changes from being liquid to solid and a blood clot (or thrombus) is formed. The blood clot is a solid mass of protein in which blood cells are caught. The blood clot appears in blood vessels, the heart or elsewhere. If it finds its way to the heart it could be fatal.

treadmill

a walking machine used to assess, diagnose, test, and monitor heart rate, and for exercise during rehabilitation.

type A and type B personalities

Studies of stress indicate that psychological stress may contribute to heart disease. Two types of personality have been identified, type A and type B. Type A people are compulsively conscious of time and work, and never want to waste a minute; type B people are more easygoing, relaxed, and less compulsive. Although the influence of personality on heart disease is not settled, it appears that type A personalities have a greater risk of heart disease.

venae cavae

the two major veins that carry blood from other veins to the right atrium of the heart.

ventricles

two pumping chambers of the heart; the right ventricle pumps blood to the lungs, while the left ventricle pumps blood to the rest of the body.

virus

a tiny particle, difficult to detect, that can reproduce within living cells of the human body, plants and microorganisms. They cause many diseases, e.g. common colds, flu, herpes, AIDS, measles, rabies, polio.

X-rays

electromagnetic radiation of very short wavelength with great penetrating powers in matter that is opaque to light. They are used in diagnosis where the techniques of radiography and radiotherapy are needed. Because unnecessary exposure to X-rays harms living matter, great care is taken in their use.

Zocor

the brand name of simvastatin, a widely prescribed inhibitor to lower the liver's production of low density lipoprotein (LDL) and, thereby, blood's 'bad' cholesterol by 20–60%: helps raise the concentration of high density lipoprotein (HDL), the 'good' cholesterol in the blood, and reduces a type of fat in the blood (triglycerides). Other brand names of similar-acting drugs that are also widely used statins are Lipex, Lipitor and Pravachol.

Selected reading

Cooley, Denton A. & Texas Heart Institute 1996. *Heart Owner's Handbook.* New York: John Wiley & Sons. A consumer education text that discusses all aspects of heart surgery from a medical point of view and shows what medical advice can be given to people who have had heart disease or are about to be treated for it.

Gaddy, Clifford G. 1994. *Triple Coronary Bypass: A Cardiologist Tells About His and How to Prevent Yours.* Macon GA: Mercer University Press. An honestly expressed and unusual personal account by a 68-year-old cardiologist of his bypass surgery in 1992. The book was intended for his family and aims to be helpful to people contemplating bypass surgery and to encourage others to practise better health care.

Hersey, April 1996. *The Insulted Heart: Recovery from Bypass Surgery.* Melbourne: Mandarin. A personal and dramatic account of heart trouble by a woman writer who looked upon her problems as a heroic challenge and her recovery as a great personal achievement.

Hyde, Jonathon & Timothy R. Green 1998. *Understanding Heart Surgery.* Banbury, Oxon.: Family Doctor Publications. A brief, clear, well-illustrated account for the lay reader of the technical procedures involved in heart surgery; the account aims to dispel the anxiety and mystery of medical procedures, and informs British readers of where to go for additional medical advice.

Martin, Johnny 1994. *Tell It Like It Is.* Launceston, Tasmania: J. Martin. A journalist's personal tribute to doctors and nurses after a successful heart

operation and recovery in hospital. Contains many amusing stories about
how difficult and embarrassing life can be in hospital.

Staff, People's Medical Society 1995. *Your Heart: Questions You Have,
Answers You Need*. Allentown PA: People's Medical Society. The writers
cut through medical jargon and crisply answer hundreds of commonly
asked questions.

Walter, Paul J. (ed.) 1992. *Quality of Life after Open Heart Surgery*. Boston:
Kluwer Academic Publishers. This is a collection of professional studies
and opinions on cardiovascular medicine, and mainly concerns patients'
quality of life after heart surgery and rehabilitation.

Worcester, Marion C. & Goble, Alan J. 1996. *Your Life after Coronary Bypass
Surgery*. Sydney: Allen & Unwin. A brief technical account from a noted
cardiologist and the director of the National Heart Foundation of
Australia's Centre for Social and Preventative Research. The account also
lists reasons for coronary heart disease, related problems, risks, and rehabilitation, and gives clear recommendations for exercises and the future
control of diet and stress.

Index

accepting loss   99
acquisition of new skills   98, 99
advice from other patients   98
  attitude to ageing   98
  fear of surgery   98, 100
  finding medical advice   97, 98
  medical insurance   98, 101
  preparing for operation   98
  public vs private hospitals
    98–9
  seeking early advice   100
  support groups   99
  take a positive attitude
    98–101, 112
  taking it easy   99
  visiting the ICU   100
ageing   81
  longevity and   95
allergies   39
American Heart Association   ix
anaesthesia   115
  after effects of   54–5
anaesthetist   38–40, 44, 50–1,
    52

angina   9, 11, 13, 32, 85, 96,
    115
Anginine   115
angiograms   3, 5, 7, 9, 11, 13,
    25, 31, 32, 34
angiography   115
angioplasty   5, 29
aortic valve   116
appearance after operation
    54–5
Aratac   115
arrhythmia   116
arteries blocked and crumbling
    3, 5, 7, 9–13
arteriosclerosis   116
aspirin   116
atherosclerosis   116
atrium   116
autologous blood supply   117
Australian Cardiac
    Rehabilitation Association
    ix
Australian Institute of Health
    and Welfare   ix

autonomy of informants:
  lost   35–6, 37, 40, 49
  regained   69–70, 71

blood pressure   117
bypass operation   x, 117
  costs of   x
  decision to operate   27
  delayed   32, 44
  demand for   5
  details of procedure   39,
    44–6
  friends' information on   39
  informants' feelings about
    beforehand   48–52
  medical explanation of
    37–40
  quadruple   3, 31, 122
  traumatic procedure   39, 45
  triple bypass   21, 46
  see also complications

cardiac ward   8, 117
cardiologist   3, 4, 6, 25, 27, 117
  decision on operation   31,
    32, 34
  informants' preferred
    characteristics of   31, 33,
    34, 95, 97, 98
  recommends surgeon   28–9,
    30–4, 112
  relations with the informants
    32–3, 97
cardiopulmonary bypass   117
cardiopulmonary resuscitation
  (CPR)   64, 117
chest appearance after operation
  66, 84

cholesterol   2, 3, 11, 12, 21, 23,
    24, 117–18
complications:
  arrhythmia   104–6
  graft failure   102
  second operation needed
    104, 107–8
  stroke   108–9
  vein clogged   107
complications, following
    operation in hospital:
  blood allergy   62
  loss of blood   61, 62
  loss of taste   73
  lung collapse   62–4
  numb foot   63–4
  pain of laughing   73
  shoulder pain   63
complications, following
    recovery at home:
  minor   102, 112
  serious   102–9, 112
codeine   118
collateral blood vessels   118
coronary angioplasty   118
coronary arteries   118
coronary bypass graft (bypass
    operation)   118
coronary heart disease   118
coronary occlusion   2, 25, 118

deep vein thrombosis (DVT)
    118
defibrillator   119
diabetes   21, 49, 88
diabetes mellitus   119
diet   2, 3, 12, 21, 23, 43, 112
dietician   43, 76, 77

driving a car   34, 79
drugs   54, 58, 65
duration of operation   56
dying:
  as an alternative   112
  experience of   8, 26, 64
  informants' fear of   46–8
  rescued from   90
  risk of   48, 68
  and the surgeon   28, 109

eating after operation   73
ectopic heart beats   119
electrocardiogram (ECG)   5, 9, 11, 119
endorphin   119
endotracheal breathing tube   119–20
  see also respirator tube
exercises   76–7, 79–80, 112–13

family of informants:
  effect of heart disease on   2, 3
  shocked by sight of informant after operation   54, 56
  visits ICU before operation   40–1
family history of informant   2, 21, 22–5
friends help informants   64, 76

haemodialysis   120
heart:
  normal functions   14–17
  in trouble   17–18
heart attack   2, 5, 7–9, 11–12, 112–13, 120

heart disease:
  and ageing   2, 20
  anxious about   2, 5, 7
  and beriberi   23
  breathing problems   3, 4, 12, 34
  causes and characteristics   x, 1–13, 18–19, 111
  chest pain and discomfort   4, 6–8, 12
  dizziness   3
  giving up on life   7
  indications from informants   21–6
  indigestion   2, 4, 7, 12
  lack of enthusiasm   13
  long-term signs   10–14
  neck pain   34
  short-term signs   x, 1–10, 14
  shoulder pain   8
  signs of   112
  sleeplessness   2, 3
  stress   3, 7, 11, 22–4
  sweating and clamminess   3, 7, 34
  throat discomfort and pain   5–6
  tiredness   2, 5, 7, 10, 13
heart-lung machine   39, 44–6, 120
heart rate   53, 56
heparin   120
hepatitis   120
hospital:
  admission to   36–7
  amusement during recovery   36
  barber's advice   39

becoming a patient in   35–6
chaplain available   38, 39
exercise and rehabilitation in
    76–7
informants' view of   32–3,
    37
information on operation
    from   37, 39
preparation for entering
    35–6
preparation for the operation
    42–3
regime takes over   37, 51
single private vs public ward
    47, 71–3
useful items in   35–6
hypertension   120–1

infarct, infarction   121
informants   ix–xi, 1
    experiences of   2–13, 21–6,
        112
    feelings about heart disease
        ix, 1
    preparing for operation   xi
    self-diagnosis and
        self-treatment   1–4, 6–9,
        12–13, 112
infusionist   121
insurance (medical)   ix, 36–7,
    98–101, 103
intensive care unit (ICU, SICU,
    ITU)   8, 11, 12, 53–60,
    121
    informants' family visits
        41–2
    time spent in   53
irritable heart   62

left anterior descending arteries
    121
legal and informed consent for
    authority to operate
    40–1, 121

mammary artery   45
medical advice on heart disease:
    explanation of diagnosis
        9–10
    importance of   xi, 1–3, 5–6,
        8–10, 13, 25–6, 112–13
    problems in diagnosis   4,
        6–8, 13
mitral valve   121
myocardial infarction   121

National Health Service (UK)
    ix
National Heart Foundation   ix,
    76
nil orally   43, 121
Nitrolingual   5, 85, 121
nurses   51, 59

oesophageal reflux   7, 122

pain management after
    operation   28, 49, 54,
    59–60, 65–6, 80, 97
panadol   122
pericarditis   122
personal life affected variously
    by operation   81, 113
    alienation   82
    concentration, mental skills,
        and abilities   80, 81, 87–8
    creativity   81, 87, 88

dependency   87, 90–1
depression   82, 87–90
drugs   89
embarrassment   82
eyesight   89
golf vs tennis   86
lifestyle changes   83–6
new active life   86, 88, 114
physical weakness   82–8
self-confidence   82, 90
shortness of breath   85
speech   88
stress   84
vulnerability   82, 87–8, 90
physiotherapist   38, 62, 63, 122
breathing technique   68–9
walking support   69–70
pulmonary arteries   122
pulmonary embolism   11, 122

quadruple bypass   122

recovery at home   x–xi, 76–80
anxiety about   80
attitude towards   77–8, 81
Ayers Rock test   92, 98
bodily signs of   94
cholesterol levels   78
community help for   94
confidence in   8
counselling for   77
discussion about   77
dressing   77
exercise classes   76–7
exercises   77, 79–81, 92
fishing   94
gardening   96
golf   81

home renovations   92
housework   61, 94, 97
meditation   78
non-smoking   77
nutrition and diet   77–9, 81
with others   76
preparation for   77
self-sufficiency   94
shopping   77
swimming   78, 79, 95
tennis   80–1
tests and challenges   92–5
vacations and holidays   92, 94
recovery in hospital—early days:
awareness of subconscious life   58–9
bruises   65
discomfort of respirator tube   57
embarrassment   65
family attitude to   54, 58, 65–6, 112
hallucinations   65
nausea   65
thirst   5
recovery in hospital—last days   73–4
food and entertainment   73, 100
going home   74–5
showering alone   73–4
visitors   71
recovery rate:
affects others   113
anxiety about future   97
attitude to   95–7
changing character of   96

compared with others   96
and longevity   95
and medical advice   113
rehabilitation programs   x,
    76–80, 93
respirator tube   46, 53
    discomfort of   59
    removal of   58
    warning about   38, 49
    see also endotracheal breathing
    tube

saphenous vein   122
showering after operation   73–4
shunt   123
smoking   2, 3, 10–11, 21–3,
    85–6, 98
staples and stitches   46
stent   123
surgeon:
    confidence and trust in   27,
        30, 32, 40, 48, 97, 98, 111
    decision to operate   27–8,
        32, 111
    informing the patient   27–8,
        33, 38–40, 89, 97, 100
    jokes with   28–9, 50
    at the operation   50–2
    paying   31

preferred characteristics of   28,
    30, 32–3, 38–9, 98, 111–12
relations with informants
    28–34, 96, 112
systemic veins   123

tests   4, 6, 11, 12
transition ward   56
treadmill   2, 5, 25, 28, 30, 34,
    80, 123
tubes in body after operation
    46, 53, 58
    painful removal of   67–8
type A and type B personalities
    123

venae carvae   123
ventricles   123
virus   124

waking in discomfort   57–9
weight   2, 11
wires in body after operation   46
women's breast discomfort   31
work, returning to   81–3, 91

X-rays   124

Zocor   2, 12, 124